THE CONFIDENCE BOOK

(How to stay sane in a world gone mad!)

By the Rogue Hypnotist

Disclaimer: the Rogue Hypnotist accepts no legal liability for the use or misuse of the information contained in this book. People who are not qualified professionals use the information at their own risk. This book is intended solely for entertainment and educational purposes. The ideas and 'exercises' are for your personal learning; copyright free. They may not be resold.

Note: British English spelling and punctuation conventions are generally used throughout. What appears as 'bad grammar' is often hypnotic language. Any repetition is by design...

Also in this internationally bestselling series...

How to Hypnotise Anyone - Confessions of a Rogue Hypnotist.
Now in French: Comment Hypnotiser N'importe qui: Les Confidences d'un Hypnotiseur Rebelle.
Mastering Hypnotic Language - Further Confessions of a Rogue Hypnotist.
Powerful Hypnosis - Revealing Confessions of a Rogue Hypnotist.
Forbidden Hypnotic Secrets! - Incredible confessions of the Rogue Hypnotist.
Wizards Of Trance - Influential confessions of a Rogue Hypnotist.
Crafting Hypnotic Spells! - Casebook confessions of a Rogue Hypnotist.
Hypnotically Deprogramming Addiction - Strategic confessions of a Rogue Hypnotist.
Hypnotically Annihilating Anxiety - Penetrating confessions of a Rogue Hypnotist.
Weirdnosis - Astounding confessions of a Rogue Hypnotist.
The Force of Suggestion part 1: Foundations.
The Force of Suggestion part 2: Changing Perceptions.
The Force of Suggestion part 3: Trojan Horses.
Persuasion Force Volume 1: Everyday Psi-Ops.
Persuasion Force volume 2: Alchemical Persuasion.
Persuasion Force volume 3: Invasion of the Mind.
How to Manipulate Everyone - level 1: Exposing the Mind Benders.
How to Manipulate Everyone - level 2: Defend Your Mind!
How to Manipulate Everyone - level 3: Taking Control!

A Warning to the Curious!

This book contains many powerful, potentially transformative ideas. You may find that in the weeks, months, and years to come that your life begins to improve in an almost astounding way that surprises and delights you. But there is a price: you cannot go back to being who you weren't. Erm…also I use swear words, sometimes: please forgive me, but they are necessary.

Are <u>YOU</u> ready?

PREAMBLE 1: ARE YOU CONFIDENT NOW?

How confident do you feel now? Make a mental note - just get the gist of it. As you go through this book and begin the process of learning to be that confident person that you really are, I want you to notice exactly when you start to feel more and more confident. If you take the tips from this book that seem of relevance to you, add in a few of your own learnings, which you're sure to make, I am confident that The Confidence Book will boost your confidence. The number 1 Key to Confidence Tip (KTC) is this - ***confidence is inevitable when you feed yourself with a diet of good information.*** There are so many of these KTCs in this book you won't be able to consciously track them. They'll become part of the background...

PREAMBLE 2: THE CONFIDENCE DELUSION.

Okay. Before we take a step further we have to get something straight. Real deep-seated confidence is not a passing, fleeting feeling, it is a state of being. In this book you are going to acquire something I call **<u>DEEP CONFIDENCE</u>**. That is, you don't *feel* real confidence, you simply ARE confident. I used to help people feel confident. Hypnotherapy for confidence works in a remedial way: it can get you back on your feet, calm you down etc. And it works, until you come up against a profound crisis of historical proportions. Then that dreadful fear comes back etc. In this book you'll learn the secrets of deep confidence: confidence that never leaves you. Some self-help 'gurus' swear that doing a couple of visualisations and 'positive thinking' will give you confidence. I am confident that's bullshit. So-called 'positive thinking' in a volatile, dangerous milieu is not going to help you. Only 100% realistic, sane thinking will help you. Thoughts are not graded as though they were types of electrical current.

PREAMBLE 3: BEFORE WE GO ANY FURTHER...

With your permission I'd like to thank your subconscious mind for doing what it did. For making you feel, believe, and act the way it did. It had its reasons, it did it all very well. *Now, I'd like to speak to YOU, the subconscious mind...Thank you so much for looking out for this person. But now, you know, it's time to change. Now you know it's time to make this person feel very confident indeed. And then some...I am your guide through this powerful change process. Please only take on the ideas, attitudes, beliefs and feelings that suit this unique person best. They don't need to know or remember how what was done, was done...it will all become just part of the 'scenery' as it were...YOU can feel confident about that.*

A CONFIDENT INTRODUCTION.

This book is needed. Great masses of people are currently overwhelmed with needless anxiety. The brain does not work optimally when it's stressed. Stress stops you from having fun. Stress stops you from laughing more often. Stress stops you from solving problems much more easily. Stress makes you worry. Worry then makes you more stressed. The solution to this downward spiral is what we call, for brevity, and convenience's sake's CONFIDENCE!

Now, let me be crystal clear at the start - there is no such thing as confidence. You can't pick it up and put it in a box. The feeling of confidence is a state of mind-body that is highly useful. But feelings pass. You need to *be* confident. A truly confident person is simply calm whilst everyone else panics. This is why we like leaders who are calm in a crisis. You can generate a temporary confident feeling, or more feeling-confidence, if you prefer, in a number of ways. One of which is through hypnosis, or hypnotherapy, if you think there's a difference. But there's another problem with hypnotherapeutic 'solutions': it can create 'confidence monsters'. *<u>The problem is: what I mean by 'confidence' and what you mean, and what he, she, and everyone else and their dog may mean by that word spell could be diametrically opposed to one another. The word is so vague it's meaningless, but useful, sometimes.</u>*

You see as a hypnotherapist I noticed something - about 93%ish of my clients were greatly helped by what I called a confidence boost sessions. However, to my lasting regret, I seemed to have made a number of people simply more arrogant than they were previously. Arrogance is not confidence. Being conceited is not confidence. Deep confidence is much more laid back, more whole, more down to earth, far more powerful. You'll learn about this.

I am going to say this now: if you are a bad person, you don't deserve to be confident. In fact fuck you for reading my book. If you are a mean, selfish, horrible person nothing in this book of resources for the truly deserving will work for you - ever. If you have personally made the world a worse place for other people YOU GET NOTHING! Are we clear?

The information in this book only works for basically kind, ethical people, not perfect people, but good, decent folk. I want to help this type of person rediscover their confident birthright. The fact is its those very bad people that rob nice people of their confidence. For fun I call the bad people 'the hell bound'. But like any thief, what they briefly stole, you can get back. You see your golden confidence is there already: its just waiting for you to uncover it. Like a diamond waiting to be discovered in the earth. You've had glimpses of it, haven't you? Under that swirling tension, those confused doubts, that sticky fear: your confidence is sitting there, looking at its watch, waiting for you to turn up and get back to the glorious adventure of living fully and joyfully, even in the midst of chaos. Not everyone can thrive during the chaos, *you will*.

Everyone is here for a deep purpose. This is a test. Your purpose is totally different from any one else. You are here to do a series of things that are important and meaningful to you, and you alone. When you re-access your confidence you will just know what these things are. If you haven't yet found that out, yet. When you do discover **the core you**, meaning and purpose will explode joyfully every day, for the rest of your life. You'll be genuinely happier, you'll feel a knowing calm, no matter what crazy shit is going on around you. You'll see the funny side of grim things. You will endure, overcome and flourish. And how do I know this? I know this because I know about people. I know that people are so much more than they have been taught to believe. If you are going to be confident, you are going to have to take off those chains that have been weighing you down. Those chains were only fairy stories anyway. It's time you stop believing in fairy stories; especially when they are told by bad witches and wizards. So if you are ready, and if you're willing. I know your are. Dive in - bravely. Don't look back. You are about to discover, if you haven't already - WHO YOU REALLY ARE! Have you ever seen a flower begin to bloom in the spring?

I confidently predict that if you simply allow yourself to easily absorb the ideas in this book, and only the ideas that seem to resonate with you at a deep, instinctive level, ignore anything you disagree with, I throw out lots of ideas to see what sticks, then your future looks bright. It looks very bright indeed. And don't be too surprised about the ways that this change manifests in reality. When you're in touch with reality you are rarely surprised.

WHO IS THE ROGUE HYPNOTIST?

Okay, once more, with feeling…The 'Rogue Hypnotist' is the pen name of a person who writes far too many books about things he knows some stuff about. This successful mad typing habit started whilst he worked as a highly successful NLP Master Practitioner and Clinical Hypnotherapist in London England. Annoyed at the lack of decent therapy training that got clients fast results this Rogue Hypnotist person created his own therapy system called, jokingly, 'Roguenosis'. For no other reason than that it sounded a bit cool, and he thought it would help him sell books. What this approach was in practise was the study of everything that worked from any system of therapy and any 'therapist' or 'hypnotist' who's methodology made sense and actually delivered results. I ended up by successfully helping most of my clients in one, one hour session 99.9% of the time. But you have to be willing. Are you willing?

Those who had received prolonged trauma and abuse took a bit longer. Prolonged trauma produces a hiding response. Trust in self and others must be reconnected to. Also some people are programmed to have an 'I can't' meta-attitude. Well fuck that shit because you were born to be an 'I can' kinda person. Prolonged brainwashing needs a bit more of a 'bash' to unglue. But, when the trust recovering brain sees that the more confidence (the more you) it releases, the better you seem to be doing in general, the unconscious 'it' just, eventually, lets the flood gates open. And when it does, and when you, each and both of you do, you'll find that that's when the magic just starts to happen, to flood in and out.

You're whole life changes. For the better, and you don't even need to know how and why. But one thing I know, and I mean really know, is that with your renewed, revivified confidence you will enjoy the ride a whole lot more.

Okay, so I've written 20, including this one, books on NLP, hypnosis, hypnotherapy, 'mind control', weirdnosis, cultural hypnosis, cults, programming, deprogramming - you name it, too many things. They all became very successful. My first very successful book was **How to Hypnotise Anyone**. I created that nearly 10 year ago. It still sells well. But, by far my most successful books are the **How to Manipulate Everyone** series, especially level 1, Exposing the Mind Benders. This is the most successful book I've written, it is so explosively popular in the United States that I am quite gob-smacked and humbled. The British haven't quite worked out what's going on yet. Slow learners. There is no more time to be slow...

All my books get to either number one or two in the hypnosis charts on Amazon.com and .co.uk. Where I publish all my works exclusively. If I publish a book it goes to the top of the charts because I actually know what I'm talking about. They are somewhat, shall we say, controversial.

I stopped writing to learn CGI (Computer Generated Imagery) for two years. I'm setting up an independent film studio. But then certain things happened, did they not, to all of us, and I brushed off my old boxing gloves and stepped back into the ring. I shit on fear. I shit on fear-mongers. You are here to get back your confidence, or maybe just for the experience. You will certainly have an experience. I'll promise you that. You need not have read any of my other books - this one stands on its own.

By the way, and this should give you confidence in me, if you are new, if you are - welcome: I mainly helped people with anxiety and addictions problems. My therapeutic expertise is in calming down the brain, without drugs, in removing unwanted habits and yes, in boosting people's confidence. A good old confidence boost is part and parcel of every hypnotherapy session. But more importantly, *I know what's going on*...You are in safe hands - this is not my first barbecue!

THE STRUCTURE OF CONFIDENCE.

The helpful myth we call confidence has, I believe, the following structure:

1. **Physical confidence:** this encompasses body language, the way you dress to express your confident self, your body shape, fitness etc.
2. **Psychological confidence:** the intermingling of your confident thoughts, attitudes, beliefs, 'life of the imagination', feelings and sensations, intuitions, insights, and instincts.
3. **Financial confidence:** having enough money, resources etc. to maintain confidence over time in order to get basic and higher order needs met.
4. **Skills confidence:** a level of expertise at X, or the doing/performing of X. X being a skill, trade, profession, knowledge on a given subject/s etc.
5. **Success confidence:** the level of consistent success in the achievement of desired goals over time. The ease with with you attain goals.
6. **'Spiritual' confidence:** how deeply you have achieved a 'oneness with the 'soul' or core of who you are. May not necessarily be connected to any religious/creed/belief system etc.

These 6 factors add up to what I call: ***THE CONFIDENCE MATRIX.*** In this book you will learn how to build your unique confidence matrix. I promise.

NO NEED FOR HYPNOSIS.

I can't formerly 'hypnotise' you, obviously. I'm here, and, well, you are there....Don't worry. You don't need a hypnotist to smash you into a deep state of hypnosis to become more confident. That's one way to do it. Kind of archaic in the current times but...Now, I might be employing a little bit of light trance tricks, now and again, but this book is talking to all parts of your brain. The conscious and unconscious. And the whatever. Then unconscious cooking occurs and voila! I have personally found the best way to be confident is to snap out of pathological trance and to join the party known as reality.

Fortunately, an idea alone is quite a hypnotic thing. Hypnosis is just a state of absorption. You ever watched a film that you really got into? That's hypnosis. The whole of reality became just that fascinating thing for two hours or so, didn't It? You forgot about everything else...for a while. You're emotions seemed far easier to access in that state. In a highly focused state we absorb information without questioning it. The talky bit of the brain takes a back seat for a bit. Thoughts drift off like bubbles in the breeze. Sometimes you need that critical bit, sometimes it needs a rest...to wonder and wander. In some situations you want the critical bit. You want it to be there to protect you from unwanted influence. You need it to examine problems and to check that your solutions are working, that you are on track. And then there's daydreams...

We go into varying hypnotic states on a daily basis. In and out. Up-...and all the way down...The most common one is when we *go into a light trance* and ponder things. You need to be lightly self-hypnotised to go into trance. Which is easy and natural. You don't need trance to be hypnotised. You can have your eyes fully open and be fully hypnotised. But, its nice to get lost in a pleasant reverie of some kind, is it not? You can fantasise about anything and everything. It's like a waking dream. When you are involved in anything at all that requires concentration you go into a kinda waking trance. All distractions melt, dissipate, and disappear. When you enjoyably focus in like that, you'll find the task is easier to complete. Tasks become more joyous, more enriching, somehow. You focus in whilst you read. Especially if its interesting. Its enjoyable to pay attention to something that's enjoyable. How funny that the arrangement of certain shapes have meaning...Confident people find it far easier to go into pleasant flow states. When *you're in trance,* you can gain access to that part of you that solves problems in highly creative ways. Solutions just seem to pop into your head when you least expect. Your instincts and intuitions just effortlessly emerge and let you know that which you really need to know. Of course that means you have to be willing to notice, listen, and take action. A confident person makes the things that they want more of in their life happen. A confident person takes responsibility.

Since ideas are hypnotic, that means the mere experience of experiencing new ideas can have a hypnotic effect. Whatever that means. There will be many ideas within this book - your book of confidence. Some will resonate more for you at differing times in your development. And that's fine too. Some might not resonate at all. That's fine also. You are in charge of this...For you, the actor in this tale, are designing in your own version of 'confidence'. I have my ideas, but they're there only to stimulate you. It's most important to me that this changing experience is yours and yours alone. For who can teach another who they were really, and I mean really meant to be? I don't even know what 'teaching' means, but one thing I have a few ideas about is how we learn, and I mean really learn, now...

HOW WE REALLY LEARN ER, STUFF.

<u>We learn best when something is important to us.</u> We learn best when we learn that which we NEED to learn. We want to learn things that help us and others improve in some way that has meaning to us and us alone. Information that you want to learn, skills that you want to learn are out there. You just have to find the things you want to focus on. Habits alter when we go toward the new habits with intent. We set goals, create ways to achieve them, and put new behaviours, or useful older ones into action. Then we check to see if we got what we wanted. We check to see that the results now and in the future are better...

Now, how do you, does anyone learn to *feel* confident? Can you learn about feelings? Can you have more of a particular feeling? Of course you can. Because your deeper mind controls feelings and can make you *feel more confident easily*, whenever you wish. But before we get to that, you need to know that the construct we call 'confidence' requires a tool set too. The tool set will lead to more confidence, in fact the tool set is confidence. And that 'tool set' is simply a bunch of new attitudes, or perhaps old ones that weren't quite as habitual as they might be...until now...The fact is that attitudes change minds. And you have a mind, do you not?

But, and yes, my friends there's a but. Every fairy story has a villain. The villain of the fairy story is, are, 'the fear-mongers'. Those who monger fear. Fearmongers come in all shapes and sizes. They are simply those who seek to make you shrink from being all that you are, and were meant to be. The world is full of slave-minded, jealous people. They want to drag you down to their cowardly level. Because if you become the hero in your own story, you point out in sharp contrast the poverty of the fear-monger-mindset. Fear, unnecessary fear, is elicited to keep you in your place, as unpleasant, unworthy others see it. The lesson I want you to take from this is: from now on *you define your place*. As all fear-mongers are liars: why would you listen to a liar?

When we learn in the traditional way we start off consciously and clumsily, maybe even with a bit of nerves. That's fine. Confident people can tolerate a bit of nerves. But that's only one way, the best way is to absorb best practise through osmosis. If you are trained by a master craftsman you just pick up his or her best practise by merely being exposed to them doing what they do, really well. It's the most magical way of learning. You can just do things without knowing how. What is magic, a deeper magic, anyway?

Now a word on nerves my friend. Nerves can actually make you perform better in a number of fields. You just want them to be manageable. You don't want life without excitement. They can make a performance in public more energetic, more passionate. However, in many situations you can get rid of nerves by taking that old, unhelpful pressure off of yourself. You see, if you demand too much, too soon, you'll demoralise yourself. You can't be great at something, anything without any practise. Funnily enough you can take pressure off by permitting yourself to make mistakes, to fuck things up, to not be perfect. Aiming at being perfect on day one is going to put a whole lot of pressure on you. Based on a delusion. The idea that - anyone is perfect, and that you should be perfect at something new on day one. Give yourself permission to be crap at first. Its liberating. You'll get better quicker. It's a paradox. But it works. Do stuff, try stuff out, have a sense of humour when you fuck up. Be kinder to yourself. See what actually works. Learn…Learn your own way of learning…

THE DEFINITION OF CONFIDENCE.

You can't become something that you can't vividly picture. Is a confident person like a lion or a mouse? Is a confident person too scared to say what they really think? Does a confident person hesitate to take calculated risks? Does a confident person walk with good posture, facing forward, arms swinging in a relaxed way by their side? Or do do they have a head that juts out like a turkey? The neck bones stretched forward, the shoulders hunched, the arms tight and constricted in their movements? You need to be aware of differences to be confident.

Confidence is literally having faith in yourself. People can lose that faith for all manner of reasons. You might lose a job. You may have experienced a trauma. You may feel your life isn't progressing as you'd hoped. You might be surrounded by confidence sapping people. ENERGY VAMPIRES!!! On my! You may have recently lost a loved one. In some way you may just generally feel things are out of control - your control that is. Someone may have betrayed you, and you now find it hard to trust. You may have made a bad decision based on bad information, and you now don't trust your own judgement. Whatever the reason, and there are many, and they are valid, however, the fact is a truly confident person can take the ups and downs of life. No one's life is wonderful all the time. Shit happens, life happens. What you want, what you can have is *confidence that endures.* You came to the right place for this. Because that place is already within you...

Now, a confident person is relaxed, yet alert. They feel no pressure to conform because the masses do. A confident person has a firm set of ethical principles, and lives by them, no matter what. A confident person takes action to make the things they want to have more of, happen - they are enterprising. They don't wait around for others to come and spot them, save them etc. They are doers. They are the dreamers who dare to dream. And in dreaming doing...

Confident people are their own experts - the buck stops with them. Confident people are independent-minded people who can think for themselves. All confident people are individualists. Even when everyone else is losing their shit, a confident person is calm. The confident person is honest but smart enough to know who they can be fully open with. A confident person creates strategies to get what they want. They try them out. If it works, great, if it doesn't - you go back to the drawing board and try something else. Smart, confident people *have a quick learning curve.* If you keep doing the same dumb thing and it's getting you nowhere...If you keep listening to poisonous advice despite the fact that it doesn't get you the results you truly, deeply want then your learning curve is too...damn slow. You need to wise up, fast. Its time to stop time wasting.

There's more to this. Look, I've said in my other books, the masses are trained by the system to learn in a linear way. To succeed in life, at life, to pass THE test, you need to make lots of connections quickly. And you can. You were born like it. Your brain is able to link lots of seemingly unconnected stuff at the unconscious level and present it to you in consciousness as a quick, surprising insight. It can do all this if you de-clutter and clear all the **chickenshit programming** out of your head. It's time...I fear, to give the finger...to the fear.

THE ATTITUDES OF A CONFIDENT PERSON 1.

Confident people own these core attributes, I call it the **CONFIDENCE MANIFESTO:**

1. They know what they want.
2. They know they deserve what they want.
3. They like themselves.
4. They have high standards.
5. They expect to be treated with respect.
6. They know who they are.
7. They do not let fear control them.
8. They have an independent mind.
9. No matter how things change, they maintain core confidence.
10. Confident people are generous.
11. Confident people have a CAN DO attitude.
12. Confident people are idealistic but practical - if they want change, they make it happen.
13. Confident people know what they're capable of: their limitations, imperfections, strengths, talents etc.
14. Confident people take risks.
15. Confident people experiment.
16. Failure is no big deal; it's something to be accepted and learnt from.
17. Confident people accept responsibility for what they have done. They do not accept blame for what they haven't personally done.
18. Confident people are generally healthy, but know when to have

fun.

19. Confident people do not blindly accept the orders or advice of so-called 'authority' figures. The main authority figure for a confident person is themselves.
20. Confident people trust their own observations and experiences over dominant, 'authorised' beliefs.
21. A confident person works on improving their faults. Weaknesses can be turned into strengths with persistence.
22. Confident people know they're not perfect but accept themselves.
23. Confident people dress well, and present themselves well - confident people are classy.
24. Confident people care about others, but they do not necessarily care what others think. Or think they think. Or thought they thunked...
25. Confident people are not jealous over other people's success. Rather they see it as an inspiration. Or they simply aren't bothered or impressed.
26. Confident people ignore rude people.
27. Confident people never let anyone steal their energy.
28. Confident people can teach themselves anything.
29. Confident people are 99% YES people.
30. Confident people see a challenge, accept it and find ways to surpass it.
31. Confident people never let the prejudice's of others affect them.
32. Confident people try to do good in the world; they try to make their world a better place.
33. Confident people have a good sense of humour.
34. Confident people have compassion.
35. Confident people are nobody's fool.
36. Confident people do not shit on others to get to the top.
37. Confident people want everyone good to succeed.
38. Confident people think outside the box.
39. Confident people are attractive and know it.
40. Confident people don't bully others or exploit or use others.

41. Confident people help others who deserve it.
42. Confident people are good judges of character.
43. Confident people judge others but are not judgemental or hypocritical.
44. A confident person is not self-righteous.
45. A confident person sticks up for the people who can't stick up for themselves.
46. A confident person has their own world view.
47. A confident person can analyse a situation accurately.
48. A confident person will listen to wise advice from wise advisers but ultimately makes up their own mind.
49. Confident people are generally happy most of the time, no matter how things change.
50. Confident people can defend themselves from attack.
51. Confident people are self-reliant.
52. Confident people enjoy the journey and the result.
53. Confident people surround themselves with genuinely supportive allies.
54. Confident people are not people pleasers.
55. Confident people are accepting of all emotions but are not controlled by them.
56. Confident people keep their head whilst the majority lose it.
57. Truly confident people do not fear death.
58. A confident person will not violate a principle of conscience.
59. A confident person is free, they would rather die fighting an evil, than live like a slave.
60. Confident people are *very* courageous.
61. On matters of core principle, confident people never give up.
62. That said, confident people know when something isn't working and can change tactics, goals, beliefs, strategies etc. when that is what is required: confident people are realistically flexible.
63. Confident people are 'first timers'; they are not fazed by accomplishing things that no one else has ever done - they think, "Oh well I'll be the *first* one to do X then."
64. Confident people don't let success go to their heads, they stay down to earth.

65. Confident people are mature.
66. Confident people choose worthy goals.
67. Confident people follow their hearts.
68. Confident people are in the main loving rather than hateful.
69. Confident people are fun to be with.
70. Everyone can be confident.

I could go on, but you get the idea I hope. As you ponder these things, as you **simply absorb** what you need without knowing how it was that each and both of you really did absorb this, you'll find the mere exposure to such ideas begins a highly positive transformative process, now, and an end…and a beginning…are all the same, are they not? Sleeping minds reconfigure things.

And even if you notice noticing some things I'm doing…because you are perceptive…it all works just the same - so relax, take a look…and continue to process this…at some level of awareness. Some people find that reading this book 3 times helps things stick. Daydreams, sleep, unconscious cooking can do the rest. You ever put some ingredients together? Suggested by a recipe and created something wonderful whilst you were off doing something else?

THE 'ASYLUM-SYSTEM' WANTS YOU TO BE SCARED.

You live in what I call the 'Asylum-System': the lunatics have taken over the asylum. The system, the system, the system. Hang on, what exactly is 'the system'? The system can be defined as the governing principles by which a given society is governed. This 'thought system', which is created by a given ruling class and their minions at any point in history is there to maintain the 'status quo'. That is 'it', 'the system', is fabricated to keep the ruling class in place permanently. To prevent genuine change in a society you must psychologically disable your opponents. A dominant minority's opponents are yes, competing systems created by other ruling classes, but the main 'enemy' to all rulers is the ruled. The ruled have to be 'kept in their place'. The ruled mind rules the ruled body.

All demoralising of the masses in society is done to create mass fear. When you are afraid your mind does not work properly. When you perceive a threat, real or fabricated your mind intensely focuses in on it. The highest material protocol of what we call the 'unconscious' mind is to keep you alive. Your brain prioritises attention and energy to mere survival functions. It releases hefty doses of stimulants - adrenaline most famously, to prepare you for fight, flight, or freeze. A scared person is so easy to control. A scared person is not free.

All human societies consist of rulers and ruled. If human society is to move forward this must end. The sheep must stop following insane leaders. Self-appointed leaders tell you they have all the answers - you're just too dumb. Your self-appointed leaders say society will fall apart if you don't do what you're told. You've all done what you were told your whole fucking lives and look at the shit state of Western society. That didn't work did it?! Modern Britain is, by any objective analysis, a totally dysfunctional shithole. If the USA continues on its current path, in twenty years it will not exist. Your 'leaders' have led you here. 'Here' is the lip of the gates of hell.

You see some people have decided they have the right to write YOUR story. Your story is for you to write. You will decide who is allowed in it. You will decide who are the wise, and who the sorcerers. You are the hero in your story, not that prick or prickess on TV. When you were born, you had the potential to write your own story. At some point you gave away your right to write your own story. You gave some shithead, or perhaps a number of shitheads the right to tell you who you were. To limit you with their limited definition of who you truly are. The you behind your name. The you that you are at night, when you sleep. The you that goes on beyond time. You are now going to take on this belief - *I will no longer be limited by limited people.* I will no longer be limited by the warped perceptions of the limited.

Everyone has limits; but the only way you discover what they are in this adventure we call living, is for you and you alone to find out what they are. To do that you have to discover what they are. Who you are. You must take risks, smart ones...when you do, you will feel more confident, *be* more *confident*. When you start pushing that big snowball of confidence, it just gets bigger and bigger. When you do that you'll find that it never melts. It just gets bigger and bigger and more and more well-constructed. Eventually you'll notice that that snowball has turned into an impregnable fortress which no army can assail. We are starting to construct the solid foundations of confidence. This process will be pleasant...

NERVOUSNESS AND MATURATION.

The core personality actually develops throughout life. You actually continue maturing until death. Some belief systems stop the personality developing as it should. A part of you knew that any way. 'Nervous problems' can develop when this maturing process is interfered with. Some time in the late 20s to early 30s, it can happen earlier, the human brain starts to fully mature. As it does it seeks to go past, eject, surpass failed belief systems that have held the core personality from fully 'unfolding'. The full maturation of the personality occurs when *the self examines its learned beliefs consciously*, and rejects past delusional programming. Much of what people believe to be 'their' beliefs have simply been installed by a whole host of 'programmers'. The Mind Benders as I call them. Programmers are people who believe they have a right to write your story. Life isn't played from a script by a woeful playwright. These control freaks stop the natural development of the unique human personality that you are. That everyone is. That will now stop...

This process of maturing is risky: there are lots of other programmers out there only too willing to write your script for you. Some people leave one play to be played by another play. You must *accept that you are the author of your story*. All confident people write their own story, that's only right, is it not? No matter what others say or do. Your story is your story. If you haven't yet, isn't it about time you fully take responsibility for your legacy? Because that's what truly confident people do. And you are one now. So...

YOU'RE NO MORE 'CRAZY' THAN ANYONE ELSE IS.

There is a big myth about a thing called 'mental illness' (MI). What people call MI is actually just a normal response to varying degrees and types of stress and trauma. It's a signal from the 'deep mind' that something is wrong. Like when you pull a muscle and feel pain. The deep mind responds to psychic pain with what we call 'anxiety', anxiety is brain pain. Essentially your mind-body-deep-mind-system is so shocked by something that occurred it goes on a hyper-vigilant war footing to protect you in future. Almost like a mild case of PTSD, which is an extreme type of anxiety. Anxiety problems exist on a continuum from mild to severe. This is not a book on how to treat or solve severe trauma. When trauma is imprinted on the mind it needs to be 'defused'; you can actually do this and take that energy and turn it into its opposite - a calm confidence. See my book **Hypnotically Annihilating Anxiety (HAA)**.

No, in this book we're talking about a very common, understandable thing; especially in these insane times. The ruling class of what once called the 'West' is at war with the rest of the population. This is a fact. If you can't deal or handle that reality, then stop reading now. Okay.

Madness can be defined in multiple ways: essentially it's believing in things that cannot be demonstrably proven. ***If you prefer, madness occurs when you believe in lies and act upon them AS IF they were true.*** All of the great horrors of history spring from this phenomena. This is why all true madness has an evil component to it.

A good person, who has common sense, and can think for themselves will never go bad, or mad. Everyone worries at times, everyone feels a bit nervous, even anxious at times. The point is: good fear protects us - it makes us pay attention to things that might be dangerous, when the brain is assured there is no immediate threat it calms you down. Anxiety goes up in an arc, peaks, and descends. With prolonged, persistent anxiety you start releasing a chemical called cortisol; this is linked to depression, which is simply anxiety gone mad. That is out of control. The 'depressed' person is in a perpetual hyper-vigilant state. They can't sleep properly. They have bizarre, violent dreams that wake them up. They become exhausted from this seemingly inescapable cycle. For some, if they don't get help, they will start to dream while they are awake. Some health care professionals think this is 'madness', it isn't, it's a sign of sleep deprivation. Hypnotherapy is excellent for calming the 'depressed' brain down, stopping it worrying, and re-establishing healthy habits, and a good sleep cycle (see my **HAA** also). In this book I'll teach you how to stop worrying, or at least dampen it down. More on this later. Very few people are truly mad; with true madness there is always a spiritual void. But that's another story.

You might be here because you lost faith in yourself. Nations lose faith in themselves. We live in a faithless society in the post-West. I don't necessarily mean in a religious sense, although that does play a big part in our collective lack of confidence. No, I mean confidence in Western values has collapsed. The current ruling class of the West hate, despise, and loath Christian values. <u>*I make no bones about it, when I say the core values of the ruling class of the West are now overtly inhumane.*</u>

The lack of values of powerful psychopaths should be of no concern to you and your confidence. You don't need to worry about what evil, mad people do. When you become confident again, their power will diminish. All evil power is always based on bluff and delusion. But I promise you that confidence is there within you, under the fear and doubt: as someone rather influential once said - *"Be not afraid."* No one can take your power from you, not with hurtful, deceptive words, not with the actions, not with state mandated fear-mongering. No. you cannot expect from others what they cannot give. I used to say this to my clients whose heart was broken because some stupid parent couldn't see how special they were. That was the idiot's loss. No one is perfect, but all good people are unique, no one can do what you do, in just the way you do it. If you care, then I care that you get back your confidence. Now...

If you are, however, reading this and think that evil people can benefit from this! What profit it a man to gain the whole world and lose his soul? You fuckers are going down with the sinking ship, and when it happens, and it will, I'll be their with billions of others cheering your worthless demise. Good people will often ask, "How do *they* sleep at night?" quite easily, because THEY don't have a conscience.

YOU NEED DEPROGRAMMING NOT REPROGRAMMING.

I once had a beautiful Russian woman as a client, she was clever, but a bit of a teacher's pet type. Some people think repeating what some random 'expert' told you is smart. No. Smart is not repeating, it's knowing. From experience. To get to my real point: I asked her what she thought hypnotherapy was. She smiled and said, "Reprogramming the brain!" "Nope…" I replied.

Look, if you came here for me to 'reprogram' you, then you got the whole shit-show topsy turvy. It's your programming that led you here. My job is to deprogram you. When you are debugged, your brain will work. You'll won't even write your own programs. You'll simply discover what is.

You were born with a brain that had the potential to work great! Then limited people started to make you believe that their limited world view was true. You were a little kid. What did you know? They were grown ups. Grown ups know everything - right? Wrong. Most grown ups don't know shit from shinola. Why do you think the world is now so fucked up? Because everyone's so smart? No. It's coz their all so fucking dumb. You don't go to dumb-dumbs when you want to be a smarty pants. There are too many nasty people in the world to allow anyone to stay dumb for long. Being dumb will fuck you up, and may get you killed.

WHY SELF-HELP IS A THING.

One sentence: loss of FAITH! 'Self-help' (so-called) arose due to two factors - the collapse of faith in Western Christianity, and the economic collapse of the West. That I am aware self help is not such a big thing in third world countries, because quite frankly they have bigger problems to worry about. The Western world has collectively lost faith in itself. You are in part infected by this collective self-doubt. It's not your fault, it's just the spirit, the evil spirit of the times. However you are you. As you are unique, you need no longer be infected by this atmosphere of aimlessness.

Nor do you have to 'rediscover religion' to regain faith in yourself. Look at the things that run the churches: you think they have 'faith'? In anything good?

Self-help developed in North America after the Great Depression (Napoleon Hill's Think and Grow Rich). The Great Depression was a psychological attack on Americana and all it stood for. After the Great Depression Americans became willing to let the state interfere in an unprecedented scale in economic and social life. As old patterns no longer worked the public looked to well publicised gurus who could help people navigate the new, altered world. As Americans are also much more inclined to a self-reliant mindset than other nations - self help appealed to this do it yourself success that defined America in the 20th century.

A big part of why self help became a thing was the explosion in research on scientific manipulation psychology. In the 20th century people started to realise you could 'succeed' by using 'mind tricks' on others to get what you wanted.

If 'self-help' was even what it claimed to be, you wouldn't be reading books on it. You want 'other help'. If you could have done what you wanted yourself, well, you wouldn't be here. What the term really means is that you want some expertise but you don't want to go see a therapist. I 100% support you in that. Although there are lots of genuinely nice, caring, skilled therapists, there are also some crazy, weird people out there.

I promise you this - if you do not need help to overcome a trauma, or severe depression that has gotten locked in and patterned, this book will help you. Even if you have been traumatised or can't stop worrying, this book will help you somewhat. It might get you 60 or 70% of where you need to get to. For people with no problems of 'clinical nervousness' this book may well get you 100% of where you need to get to. If we were one to one, I could tailor a hypnosis session just for you. I'd work out your problem matrix and create a solution. But I don't do therapy any more. All I can do is chuck out a huge amount of stuff I've learnt and hope that some of it helps. I think it will. You see, a truth: *__if you start going in a particular direction, certain inner motive forces start to see what your doing, and they get involved, and start to turn the whole ship wholeheartedly in that direction__*. When you focus all your heart and soul on the goal of getting some particular thing, then that is where the ship will start sailing to. You may find buried treasure there. Is there an easy way to kick start the confidence habit? Yes. You can do some physical things to free up the body and allow the new thoughts and feelings in. Let's do that right this moment.

THE PHYSICAL BASIS OF CONFIDENCE.

The following section is going to give you some tips I picked up from being a professional actor. I always used to use this little hypnotic phrase in a client session - where the mind leads the body follows, and where the body leads the mind follows. I have no real idea what this means, but it sounds brilliant.

Psychologists have their little bag of tricks for helping people. I once had a client who was permanently exhausted. He had seen a psychologist, in their expert god-ness, and sheer multiple letters after their name genius they had electrocuted this man to stop him feeling exhausted. Surprisingly, this electrocution stuff delivered zero positive results. Shocker! I 'cured' him in one session. He had grown up in a family where everyone was afraid of the father. The father had a mere presence that intimidated all who encountered him. My client said his father had never hit him, ever, but he always remembered being scared of him.

Prolonged fear is very tiring. This client of mine had created, as a young child, a deep patterned system of mechanisms to cope with living in an environment of fear. This fear, and the patterns he had created to deal with it, left him with no energy for anything else. One trick he used was the use of the word 'logical'. When I suggested an idea to him he responded by saying, "That sounds logical." This computeresque language told me this man was terrified of accessing his feelings. The bit that makes us human. In itself this would be exhausting.

Now, as fear robs you of confidence, and as fear is exhausting, I am going to show you how to rid your body of tension quickly. There are no breathing exercises involved. No visualisations. I just want you to do some things. If you do as I say, it will work. You will feel more confident, and more relaxed, yet you will not feel sluggish or spaced out as a person can after meditation, 'self-hypnosis' etc. Get ready to act differently, to act confidently.

The physicality of confidence.

You need to take on the physical characteristics of a high status confident person - someone with dignity, pride, and morals.

Please stand up. It's best to take off your shoes. Read this process, then put the book/kindle down and carry it out. Make sure you are doing this in private, if you are in public or on public transport as you do this, everyone else will think you've gone nuts.

Okay. Imagine that a piece of string is attached to the top of your head. Imagine that something is pulling it up. As you do this, your entire head and spine should be pulled up so that your head and neck are straight. This will bring your body into full alignment. If your spine is not in alignment, you cannot be confident - not actively confident. Laid back confident at times? Yes, but we want full physical confidence, now. Do this in a relaxed manner - you are not an army private on parade.

Let your hands hang by your sides, your face should be relaxed, your eyes simply looking straight ahead. Make sure your jaw is at a right angle to your neck. Your chin should not be pointing up, nor down. As you've aligned your spine, your chest should not be collapsed in. Your shoulders should be relaxed, not hunching. You trapezius muscles should not be involved. Your head is like a floating balloon pulling the whole body into the correct posture for confident living.

Make sure your buttocks are relaxed, Your feet are gently placed on the floor. Without shoes your feet can relax. Notice the feeling of the floor/ground under your feet. Your hips should be aligned with the spine. Don't tuck them back - sticking out your butt. Don't jut/pull them forward. They should be comfortably facing straight forward. Your legs should feel relaxed yet straight, no knee bend. You now have the posture of a confident person. You can keep that and readjust your body like that whenever you need. And if you do you'll feel confident, active, and easy going very quickly.

There's more.

Nervous people do things too fast. Slow the fuck down, now. Speak more slowly, take your time, enjoy taking your time. Relax your throat by opening up your throat - a simple yawn does this. You can, with your mouth closed simply become aware of the back of your throat - allow it to relax. It will naturally open out.

Move more slowly. For practise you can exaggerate, just so you can feel the difference. Lift up your arm and hand to the side like a ballet dancer - smooth and slow. Move them slowly and gracefully. Practise walking with good posture, but slowly and deliberately. Now, in real life such slowed down actions would look odd. You won't be this slow in real life. What it shows you is that - the way you use your body has an immediate and direct effect on your feelings. Tense people have fast, racing thoughts. Consciously...slow...them...down. When you think... more...slowly...you can...calm...all...the...way...down. Good. Again you don't want to do this in real life. But it shows you - the speed that you think at, affects your feelings. Are you getting the idea of what I am getting at? You have more control over you than maybe you thought. We've only just got started. So much for posture...

Exercises for shaking out the muscles.

Okay, now, there's a really good way to get rid of stress in the muscles, it's really simple. You just shake it out. Theatre actors have been doing this for well over one hundred years. Psychologists teach a relaxation technique where you clench all your muscles one by one and then let them relax. That's just retarded, and could give an already tense person a cramp. This is how you do the shake out...

We all collect a lot of tension in the neck, shoulders, jaw, and hands. Tension can go everywhere. It can collect in the legs. Thankfully you can shake that bastard out. Let's start with the hands. Simply focus on one hand, doesn't matter which. Now just shake it loosely. Just shaking it back and forth five times will start to relax it.

Now focus on an elbow. Starting that shake from the elbow shake your your forearm so that the shake travels down to the finger tips. You can raise your forearm up so that your loose hand is near your ear and then fling that out that arm to the side in a shake. Good. Repeat a few times.

Now fling out the entire arm from the shoulder. Do this a number of times. Now just let your arm rest at your side and gently wiggle it from the hand. Can you notice already that it feels less tense? Do this with both arms. You can do it to them one at a time or together. Improvise shake out moves.

Now stick your arm up in the air like you were sticking up your hand in class - stretch up, that's it. Now let that arm go floppy and drop it to your sides. Do that a few times. You can even shake it out on the downward flop if you like. Now let's do the legs and feet.

Pick a foot my friend, any foot. Hold onto something if your balance isn't so good. Simply lift that foot and shake it loosely - don't do it too fast, fast may hurt. Shake that foot out like a limp rag. Shake it back and forth, side to side if you can. By the way if *anything* hurts stop. If you're doing this right it feels nice.

Okay, when your foot feels nice and relaxed we can do the whole leg. Grab hold of something to support yourself. Simply swing that leg back and forth like a floppy rag doll, back and forth. Do that for a bit. If you like, and if it helps, you can flick out the arm or leg, as though it were a whip - as though you were flicking that tension out of that limb. Now, just shake that leg back and forth loose but quick. Your foot should be flopping around stupidly at the end. When you've shaken and flopped that leg to your heart's content, notice how that leg and foot feel more relaxed - yet you feel more alert. Confident people are relaxed and alert, not sluggish. Do the other leg.

You ever noticed that when you see confident people that their movements are assured, confident, dynamic? Confident people are effulgent - they seem to glow with confidence. If they're a person, and you're a person, you could walk around in a confident, purposeful way. Some people slouch around, without any purpose. **_A confident person moves with purpose._** They know what they want, they know where they're going. They're determined to get what they want. Challenges are there to be overcome. What accomplishment is worth anything if it isn't fought for? Confident people have doubts. A certain amount of doubts let us know if what we are doing is working. But, unlike a giver-upper, or a worrywart, a confident person never gives up.

Now back to the body shake. Standing upright - lift those shoulders...and drop them, do that a few times. Now gently shake those shoulders up and down a bit. Now, brace yourself - shake the core of your body - the torso/trunk left to right quickly, from the shoulders keeping your waist in place. Shimmy. This wiggles and shakes out the shoulders and arms.

Now, one at a time take each arm and fling it out a few times, as though you were trying to throw your hand away, but it won't come off. Good. Now, relax. How much more relaxed but alert do you feel now?

Now, time to shake that butt. You'd be surprised how tight those buns can become during stress. Raise your arms and bend them, as you would if you were pretending to be a chicken. Okay - now shake those hips left-right-left-right-left-right very quickly! Do that a couple of times. Make sure those gluteus maximus are nice and loose. Act as though your trying to shake something off you ass/arse. That's it...I just got you to shake your butt. I own you now.

Now arm swings. One arm at a time, spin those arms - swing forward as fast as you can, just like you are pretending to be a windmill. Now, spin that arm in reverse. Make sure the shoulder, arms, and hands are like floppy spaghetti as you do this.

Hip roll. Sit in a chair. Lift up your knees and drop your legs a few times. One leg at a time - roll that leg out to the side and drop it. As though you are making an arch shape leading with the knee. Now, shake the legs out. Next. Rotate your hips one way, then the other - as if you are trying to grind a hole in that chair by rotating your butt.

Neck next. Huge amounts of tension are stored in the neck. We are simply going to do a neck roll. Don't do this if you have any neck pain etc. Simply gently and floppily roll your neck in a circle five times to the right, then the same to the left - you can do this sitting in a chair, like they do at the Actor's Studio. Or you can try this method: stand up, bend your knees. With your knees bent place your hands on your thighs just over the knees. Maintain this position, kinda like your standing up and taking a crap. Don't actually crap! Now, rotate the head - five times one way, five times the other way. Good.

Now, I'm going to teach you a great stress, tension, posture, back saving exercise. I don't know if it has a name, so I'm gonna call it 'The Flop'. I learnt it in Youth Theatre. An American Actress taught me. All my best teachers were Americans. Except one. He was Scottish. This is how you do the flop: stand up straight, looking ahead - make sure you're nice and relaxed. Again don't do this if you have any serious back or neck pain. However, if you have tension in these areas this exercise will start to gently release it.

The Flop.

1. From the standing position bend your knees slightly.
2. Slowly, and I mean slowly, tip your head toward the floor.
3. Your intent is to be hanging upside down from your waist - your arms dangling at the side of your head.
4. As you slowly lower yourself down - imagine you are a liquid, pouring yourself down head first, toward the floor, one vertebrae at a time.
5. Let your arms drop and flop, hanging down limply.
6. As your spine stretches out using the weight of that big head of yours as a pulley, simply hang in that flopped over position. Notice any tension, or stiffness in that spine-neck continuum. As you continue to hang it will ease itself out. Don't do anything - let it happen.
7. Hang for a good ten seconds.
8. Now time to go back up. Do the same in reverse. Slowly, and I mean slowly, using the muscles attached to your spine, pull that head up, one vertebrae at a time. Do this until you are standing upright and relaxed. Notice any change. Do you feel more alert, opened out, generally freer? If you go back up too quickly you might feel dizzy and light-headed. If you do stare at the palm of your hand for a few seconds. If you crawl back up slowly, the dizziness shouldn't be a problem.
9. Repeat the whole process two more times. Each time you repeat this spinal column stretch you should feel less stiffness and tension. When you get good at this you can gently bounce at the bottom phase, with your arms and head bopping up and down like floppy spaghetti. However, if you are old/unfit etc. be careful. We don't want injuries. Health and confidence are linked. More on this later.

Let's focus on the jaw. People can store so much tension in those powerful biting jaw muscles. There's a simple remedy. Pretend you're chewing toffee or a big wad of chewing gum/bubble gum. Pretend you're a cow. Chew that cud on one side of the jaw, then another. Do that for about 10 seconds or so. Really roll that big blob of whatever it is you are imagining your are chewing. After we correctly exercise a muscle - it relaxes. Notice after a bit how much looser the jaw feels.

Face tension release time. Screw your face as though you are trying to make it all fit into the centre. You close your eyes. Pucker your lips. Bring that brow toward the nose. Scrunch that nose and chin. Okay hold it a bit, then release. Now it's time to make that face as wide as possible. Stretch out that big mouth really wide. Make your eyes as wide as you can. Wrinkle your forehead up. Pull those cheek muscles back. Hold it. Release. You can do those two manoeuvres two more times if it helps. Notice how much more loose your face is.

The lips - mouth tension release. Blow your lips as if you are a horse. Now do that thing you did when you were a kid and enjoyed being silly. Blow your lips really fast so they vibrate and it feels all tingly. Do it as fast as you like. Confident people don't mind being a bit silly when it's appropriate. Unconfident people have forgotten that it's okay to have fun. We need some fun in our lives. Fun banishes fear.

The second to last thing to do is yawn. Pretend to yawn - exaggerate it. Feel the back of your throat open up wide. This helps get rid of throat tension. Do that a couple of times - fake exaggerated yawns.

The last tension buster I get from the Actors Studio. It involves crunching your 'shoulder blades' (actually the big triangular-shaped trapezius muscles) to get rid of back tension. It really works. A complete dick-head from the Actor's Studio taught me it. But it works, so: you can do this sitting in a hard chair, or standing, either way works. Raise both hands up in the air, at the side of your head. Now, leading with those elbows. Pull those elbows down toward your waist - but toward the back - pushing the traps against one another, then raise those arms back up - again, pushing the traps together. As you do this you should feel those trapezius muscles pushing against each other. Do this a couple of times more - arms up, then pull down and back, then arms up again etc. - aiming to scrunch those big trap muscles together. Now relax and jump up and down on the spot to shake out tension all over. Shake your head so all the flesh is floppy - be careful. Now all that is done - notice how much more relaxed yet alert you feel. This is how a confident person feels.

You can do these 'exercises' whenever you feel like it. In private that is! Actors do this kinda stuff before a show. It creates energised focus. But there's more...

Confident people speak out!

Quiet, timid people speak inwardly. Their head and eyes go down. They mumble apologetically. Confident people speak out! OUT! OUT! OUT! Have you ever heard a little bird tweet away happily in the trees? That little bird could fit in your hand, but he chirps out proudly with his song. You must do the same - SPEAK OUT! **<u>The reason a decent person speaks to another is to connect with, to contact directly, another soul.</u>** This is why no one likes talking to a bureaucrat/functionary etc. A person who reads a script to you is not interested in a meeting of souls. They are interested in getting money from or imposing arbitrary rules on you.

To speak out you need breath support - more on this soon.

Stop fidgeting.

Nervous people fidget. They're antsy in their pantsy. A confident person is still. All great actors have a powerful stillness on stage or screen. If you catch yourself twiddling your fingers, biting your nails, chewing your bottom lip etc., be conscious of it and stop it. If you keep noticing habitual fidgets and stopping them, you'll do it less and less, then you'll stop. I could hypnotise you to do this instantly, but I can't so, you'll have to train yourself. A golden rule of self or other influence is **_you can use the physical body to get to the subconscious._** As I said, if you seriously set out in a new direction the other than conscious processes will notice your efforts and kick in to assist you.

Building in relaxation: tension spotting and releasing.

Part of an actor's training consists of learning to be relaxed. **_Tension stops the natural flow of expression and energy in the body._** A trick to try as you are building-in your new confident character is to simply notice where any tension is in your body. Do a body scan. Where do you feel tense now? Just notice where that tension is. Now release it. Stop scrunching that foot. Stop holding your body in that awkward position. You can get rid of light tension by simply noticing it, and releasing it. Shake it out if you can. Notice tension, release tension. Once you start doing this, sooner than you think, you'll be letting go of tension easily. You'll also have a physical indicator of when your stress levels are starting to edge up. You'll see the early warning signs and be able to do something to still the mind and chill before it gets out of control. Being aware of yourself is not a bad thing.

Increase your breathing capacity.

Many books on anxiety control talk on and on about breathing. They teach you what I call 'symptomatic breathing exercises'. That is, wait till you get all worked up, then start doing some little breathing rite/ritual to make it all right. Nope. Also such altered breathing can make some people more anxious still. Nervous people have a shallow pattern of breathing. You need to learn how to breath from the diaphragm, the big sheet of muscle at the base of your ribs. You need to practise being able to extend your breath capacity until you can breath out for a count of 30.

Breath capacity exercise.

1. Gently breath all the air out of your lungs. Push it out from the diaphragm, not the throat. Do so without noise - don't blow as though you are pretending to be a noisy wind. This puts tension on your vocal cords.
2. Now let that in breath occur naturally.
3. Now this time - breath out slowly, controlling that breath.
4. Notice how long you can do so - 10 seconds?
5. Repeat stages one to 4. This time: aim for 15 seconds on your out breath.
6. Do this every day for about 3-4 weeks. When you can comfortably breathe out for an easy, gentle 30 count, you have succeeded. Don't force it, let the increase happen naturally and gradually. Do the routine 3 times only per session. It should only take a few minutes to do.

After you practise this you will always have the breath support to speak out confidently. Your words won't run out of air to bounce along. You can also hum to increase your vocal strength if you like. Just gentle humming, now and again will do. Hum a tune in your voice range. Not too high or low.

Develop a regular stretching routine.

Anxious people are physically stiff and inflexible. Go out and buy a good book, or books on stretching. Develop your own stretching routine. Watch a YouTuber who teaches stretching if you're strapped for cash, or check out websites on stretching. Confident people are physically and mentally flexible. Stiff muscles can be relaxed by a regular - 3 days a week stretching routine. Stretching, good posture, shaking bits out and breathing cost you nothing but time. In time you'll feel more supple, relaxed, stronger, and more purposeful.

But this isn't enough: it'll get you started, and help maintain physical confidence, but the problem goes deeper...

CONFIDENCE SAPPING BELIEFS.

All confidence sapping beliefs start with a premise that somehow or another you just aren't 'good enough', whatever the hell that means. Good enough according to whom? Someone who doesn't like or care about you? Why would you care what such a person thought? Just because someone, whoever that may be, incorrectly or maliciously mislabels you as being 'inadequate' doesn't mean that label, that characterisation is accurate. Hateful people say hateful things. Stupid people say stupid things. Stop caring so much about what other people said or say about you. If it's not true, if their perceptions and/or intentions are warped - what do you care? It's time to stop giving a fuck!

Some parents, some teachers brainwash some children, when no one is there to protect them, that somehow, they are no good, badly made, not up to scratch. If this goes on for long enough - some children start to believe it. They get brainwashed into believing they're 'bad', when all that has happened is that you've encountered an ass/arsewipe. Anyone who tells a nice, innocent child that they are x, y, z list of 'bad' things is a truly bad person.

All the most abusive people you'll ever meet project all their own vile attributes onto those around them. People who are dead on the inside can't love. If someone evaluates you without love - stop caring what they think. They may not even have really thought it, they just wanted to upset you, to get a reaction, and get off on that reaction. ***What you have to understand is that no one has power over you unless you give them that power.*** I have a rule in life: I never take any shit from anyone. Nor should you. If people fuck with me there are consequences.

Common beliefs that unconfident people have been brainwashed to have are:

"I would like to do x, but I am just not good enough because I'm... somehow 'inadeqaute', too stupid, too nervous, blah etc."

Let me tell you something. For some reason I'd convinced myself I couldn't play a musical instrument. I accidentally self-hypnotised myself. I'd tried to learn violin at school, but the teacher was so twee and middle class, the other kids were such drips. So I gave up. Some forty plus years later my brother, who is a really great guitar player (he was offered record deals with major record industry players - and he turned them down!) said why don't you learn an instrument? I thought, well, I don't really want to, I suppose it might be nice, but...So I decided to learn the recorder, soprano recorder. Yes, that squeaky, little thing that girls play in school. I thought it's cheap and easy. Why not?

Within one year I was intermediate level in skill. I had a musical talent. I didn't know because I never tried. The only way you know what you can and can't do is to try. You don't always know what latent talents you have. I'm willing to bet that if you need this book - you don't know who you really are. You haven't had the courage to try. If I had been crap at the recorder or hadn't had any talent I would not have been crushed; I would have learnt a bit more of what I was truly capable of. What would you like to try? I dare you to do it.

What if you turn out to be good at something you never imagined you would be good at? Discovering things about yourself opens you up to new experiences. When you learn new skills it builds confidence, another string in your bow. What if you were a constant work in progress. What are you *really* fully capable of? If you fail - so what? I tried golf - I stink. I was so bad people laughed. I really don't care. Unconfident people say in their minds in a tone of terror, "What if x 'bad' thing happens!!?" A confident person says, "So what if x bad thing happens? I can use the experience to tell people a funny story." Unconfident people live in mind caves. You need to get out of the mind cave to get confidence. You need to try things. You need to write your own story.

Unconfident people often compare themselves unfavourably to others - "Oh I could never be as good as her etc.?" Okay. If you never tried, how would you know? And if you are worse than them, so what? It's no big fucking deal is it? Unconfident people make mountains out of molehills. Confident people have better things to worry about. You need to face the fact that everyone is actually good at a lot of things. Some people excel at them. I bet there are lots of things that you do a thousand times better than me. I'm not good at loads of things - the difference between me and you is: I don't give a shit. I'm very good at some things, and I'm happy with that; I know who I am. If you don't have the guts to find out who you are, no one can help you. You have failed the test.

One of the reasons we're here is to find out who we are. KNOW THYSELF. No one else can teach you that. You interacting with life teaches you that. Now, use your common sense. I once had a 'depressed' client come to see me. At the end of the session he said, "That was great, I'm going to become a male escort!" Hey, I don't want to piss on anyone's parade but I don't think ladies would pay cash to see this particular man in a thong, shaking his bits and pieces around. He might get arrested. He was a small, balding, glasses wearing lifer senior civil servant. No one wants to see his dick. This is a case of bad decisions leading to bad actions which sap your confidence. So make smart decisions to build your confidence; don't just swing out wildly at life and expect results. When you are confident, you'll just get a sense of what you should do. Under that shield of fear is you. You are a beautiful statue, waiting to be made. The artist is you.

Another limiting belief unconfident people have is, "I'd like to do x but I'm too nervous to..." STOP! Nervous? I don't care how nervous you are. Everyone is a bit nervous, nerves help you perform better. With practise you'll calm down. Actually a lot of unconfident people are 'perfectionists'. They usually have a parent who brainwashed them to be like this. With hypnosis this is easy to solve. However, I can't formerly hypnotise you. You could find someone who can. But, can I make a suggestion? When you feel those nerves, as you go after what you really want from this life, I think you feel those nerves really because you care. It's important to you. That's a good thing.

<u>When you first do something you'll do it the least successfully.</u> Like my friend when he lost his virginity. He lasted all of 30 seconds, and thanked the girl in question profusely after. Finally he'd got it over and done with. Once you've broken the ice, done the thing you wanted to do, it gets put in the brain in the 'I know how to do this stuff' section. Eventually you'll build up a whole host of skills like this that you can draw on. And its never too late in life to try something new. If the first time is the worst time, and it may not be, you may have beginner's luck, then you just need the courage to take the first step, after that all your inner motive forces become marshalled to assist you. The mind loves a unifying direction to go toward. What it hates is indecision and chaos. I don't care what you do, just do something. You need a plan? We'll get to that.

"People like me don't do that…" I would mainly get this self-pitying whine from working class clients. Working class people in Britain get brainwashed that people 'like us' don't do 'that'. 'That' being what they really want to do. Look, this isn't the Middle Ages. Some wretched people would like to turn things back to the Middle Ages, but…Look America proved the European class system was garbage hundreds of years ago. America was, and hopefully will be again, a meritocracy. It doesn't matter about other people's prejudices and delusions. It matters about you and whether you have the balls to go after what you want. It used to be called the American Dream. You need to create your own life dream. Wherever you live. But it's not a dream is it, it's your idea of 'the good life'; your life as you truly deeply want it to be. And only you can make it happen. No one is inherently better than anyone else; anyone who suggests otherwise is cleanly a person of no worth at all. Every child, from every background, has a human right, a 'God' given one to fulfil their potential. You were a child once. What dreams did you have? What disconnected you from your purpose? Who did you allow to write your story? The only author of anyone's story is the hero/heroine. The future is not set in stone, you make the future happen by your actions. Inaction is also an action. So what new confident actions are you going to take?

I had a teacher, an English teacher who said never use the word'got'. I thought, you've got to be kidding...If it helps, and if you're aware of them: write down all your confidence stealing beliefs. When you've done that, give them the finger, and chuck them in a bin/trash can.

YOU CAN'T BE IGNORANT AND CONFIDENT.

If you aren't widely read: that is, if you don't read a lot of books on a lot of differing topics you'll never be truly confident. How can you be ignorant and confident? You can't. Ah! But I know lots of stupid confident people. Yes, it is true there is none as bold as the dumb. But is a false boldness based on a total lack of comprehension of reality confidence? A slug is confident: in his slugness. I have seen plenty of stupid people swanning down the highstreet with a look of proud stupidity on their face. But they are not really confident. They're just dumb: remember the film, The Jerk, with Steve Martin when his black dad tests to see if Martin's character will be okay out in the big bad world? He tests to see if Martin knows the difference between shit and Shinola. When Martin shows he does know the difference his adopted dad says, "Son. You're gonna be alright." Lots of people out there don't know shit from Shinola. If you do, you're 90% ahead of all the other dumb fuckers out there, and that should make you *feel confident.*

You know when you have to go to the doctors? You don't feel right. You can't work out why. You worry. You go to the doctors: he, she tells you what the problem is - you relax. Why? Coz you know. **Your ignorance has been replaced by knowledge. Knowledge allows you to relax.**

Imagine you are in an air crash. You survive. You are in the wilderness, you need to make a fire until the rescue people turn up. Do you know how to light a fire in the wild? If you don't, you could be fucked. We need the right knowledge to survive.

Learning is fraught with so many perils, when you first start out, because ***you don't know what you don't know*** - you're that ignorant. The stupid can't be helped. But, we've all been in a postilion of ignorance, and we've all learned. There are many perils on the winding path of life with many hawkers calling out for us to let them write our story, as if they have the answers to all the problems there ever were or could be. If this is so, why is Western society falling apart? Do the 'wise' only produce crap?

Things are built and collapse by design. A thorough knowledge of real 'history' and real 'psychology' (by history I mean knowing what actually happened in the past, by psychology I simply mean an understanding of people) are essential to living. A knowledge of how to maintain health is essential. You should master your job or craft so that you know all there is to know about it. You should have good general knowledge. You must have good experiential knowledge. Book knowledge is all well and good. But real world stuff can't be beat. **Your main teacher should be what you actually observe from experience.**

I was watching a TV show about rookie police being trained by experienced serving officers. The police were called out to a domestic dispute: a man was attacking his wife - he was believed armed. The female rookie cop follows the veterans, they walk by a window and duck, she stays upright. Later on her supervisor tells her - never walk in front of a window with a possible armed suspect behind it! It was actually just common sense. But common sense ain't that common. Use your common sense.

Follow any trail of learning that genuinely takes your fancy: you wanna be a better cook? That's a great life skill. Not many of my weight loss client's had it. You can read, take classes, watch TV shows, YouTube etc. You can learn what you need to learn. The more you know the more confident you get. Never stop learning. Arrogant people stop learning, think they know it all, and stagnate. There is always more to know. You don't know now, what you'll know in the future. That's exciting! Are you confidently ready to know? You are part of a new generation that can have access to more information than any previously.

In order to do well you need to know about people: you need to know the difference between a real person and a psychopath. The latter are more common than most suspect. There are too many simply petty nasty people, let alone the psychos. Don't assume everyone has your best interests at heart. Learn to discern the good people from the bad: if you can develop that skill, it may be the most important, you'll become truly confident. Why? You'll stop making such dumb decisions. The aim of all confident people is to become wise. Confident people have wisdom. Develop yours, in your own way.

What I am saying in a long-winded waffly way is that **_you must become your own teacher._** As you take this new road, you'll be pleasantly surprised at where you end up, what new things you'll learn, what more thrilling things you'll do, and with whom you'll chose to do all that wondrous stuff with.

EVERYTHING INVOLVES RISK!

Almost everything we do involves an element of risk. We never have 100% control over every situation, we do have more leverage and influence than we often realise however. Confident people understand that if you want to do things that are out of the ordinary, you are going to have to take some risks. You have to make a potential cost benefits analysis. If I do x what could be the potential losses? If I do x what could be potential risks be? Sometimes you just have to say fuck it and go for it; if that's what you really want. Do not ever kid yourself that you live in some risk free world. The world is fraught with risks. But then it always has been. At one time in history man took a risks that the large animals he was hunting would kill him, but it was that or starve. Risk is a part of the process of living. Life is a gamble, but you take calculated risks. Don't bet the house and kids on red when the odds are long.

YOUR CONFIDENT VOICE.

I have already spoken about the voice and it's relation to confidence. As your body is 'you' to others, so is your voice. We all use our voice to influence others. We can also write, which is simply a visual-symbolic recording of our voice. This allows us to communicate across time and space.

A strong, confident voice requires not only breath support, it requires resonance. Resonance is created by humming which is directed toward the resonance chambers on the body - these include: the mask of the face (the muzzle/mouth), the throat, the forehead, the dome of the skull, the nose, and finally the chest. By gently humming and by directing the hum to these resonators you will increase the strength and attractiveness of your voice.

A confident voice also requires power: this comes from the diaphragm. Singing in the shower is another way to give your voice strength. Singing is good for the voice. If you look after your voice as you do your body you'll have a youthful sounding voice well into old age.

Salute to the sun exercise.

This process will give your voice power, your body will relearn how to naturally project your voice. You used to use your voice this way as a child. You ever heard a baby that doesn't know how to influence people with its voice?

1. Lie on the floor, arms at your sides, or resting on your tummy, with your knees bent, feet on the floor. This position allows the entire body to relax creating pure voice production only. You can

do this with your eyes closed, though it's not needed.
2. Gently blow out all the available breath you have - do so in a controlled way using your diagram muscle.
3. Let your lungs fill naturally.
4. With the intention to sing a song to the sun release that breath on a comfortable note using the word 'Ma!' the M projects the sounds, the A sustains it.
5. The sound should sound attractive, clear and strong.
6. Just allow the note to gently fade with your breath capacity.
7. Pick another note within your range and let out another 'Ma!'
8. Always allow the breath to happen naturally. Sing out. Let the lungs fill naturally, then sing out again when they're full.
9. Repeat between 3 and 10 Mas! On differing notes. You want vocal strength across the full range of your voice - high and low.

If you practise this repeatedly every day or even just 4 days a week for 3 weeks I promise you'll have a naturally much more confident sounding voice. Confident comes from doing things right, not hypnosis scripts. You must bite into the arse of life my friend! That's how you get confidence!

DO YOU WANT ATTENTION OR CONFIDENCE?

I think this is a fair question. You see confident people don't care about getting attention from random strangers. They're are quite comfortable in themselves. Attention seeking is a mild form of addiction. Some people get little boosts of good feelings doing it. They think that when they get attention it means others love and like them. Nope, it just means you got attention. Getting attention for? Hmmm. When you are truly confident you don't care about approval or disapproval. When you get attention, it's because you did or said something that naturally attracts people. You are not an entertainment monkey.

TRUSTING YOUR GUT.

Instincts my friend! Instincts! Confident people trust theirs. Let me tell you, **<u>a large number of people get into trouble because they do not listen to their instincts.</u>** People with weight problems fail to pay attention to the fact that their 'gut' is sending them a message, via a little image of a meal it wants them to eat. That meal would fulfil their nutritional needs. They ignore that message and eat 5 cupcakes instead. An athlete feels a niggle in his knee, ignores it, and snap, something gives. He is injured. A woman has a bad feeling about a man she is dating, ignores that feeling - she's in an abusive relationship; her gut tried to warn her, she didn't listen. She checks her black eye in the mirror.

The fact is that your unconscious processes are noticing far more than the conscious mind can. The unconscious communicates with the conscious via images, thoughts/ideas that just bubble up, often with solutions whilst you're doing something else. It sends feelings and sensations, sometimes involuntary movements of muscles that may indicate a positive or negative evaluation of a given situation you might find yourself in. All of my therapy clients, without exception, habitually ignored such signals. Listen to yours. Nervous/unconfident people ignore the guiding wisdom of the deep mind. When you pay attention to such communications you'll be calmer. Your conscious mind and unconscious mind need a good rapport. If they don't a person can start to feel in two minds. One part is pushing for one thing, another part another. This doesn't work. Confident people are aligned and congruent. Your gut is a big part of your decision-making apparatus. It even effects our morality. Ever felt that you shouldn't have done something and went ahead and did it anyway? Only to feel bad about it afterwards. Jiminy Cricket.

ALL EMOTIONS ARE ACCEPTABLE.

Confident people go through all the same range of emotions as other people do. Grief, sadness, pity, anger, rage, calm, joy, bliss etc.; all the emotions are acceptable. At times you'll feel worry and fear. But here's the thing. They all pass, they won't overwhelm you. All suffering passes. Wounds heal by degree. Confident people experience life, that means experiencing a wide range of emotions. Nothing good or bad lasts forever. Emotions rise, surge, peak and decline.

If you think becoming confident is all about only feeling 'confident' forever, you're in for a shock. Humans feel a wide range of feelings, that's what is is to be human. But you'll be in control of those feelings. And underlying even grief at a loved one's passing, is that there is always that underlying strength that a confident person has, what they gave you is within you always, and we all meet again whether you believe it or not. Under sadness there is a core confidence supporting you. You are not made of iron, you are sensitive, you have a soul. Be confident about that.

THE MYTH OF 'SELF-ESTEEM'.

It was the British philosopher David Hume who invented the idea of a 'self-esteem', until he did this in the 18th century, people had got on fabulously without one. I had clients who imagined they had low self-esteem. As this is just an imaginative construct it's very easy to get them to imagine having healthy self-esteem, which is an equally made-up schema; but it has its uses.

We all evaluate ourselves. We all evaluate others. Some people are unfortunate in that they do not grow up in families where they are loved unconditionally. Children believe that they must be somehow bad, wrong etc. if no one loves them. They are too little to realise that the fault lies with the dead on the inside parents, or evil-stepmother etc., and not with them at all. Such child rearing environments can scar the individual's evaluation of themselves: in essence they adopt the evaluative scale of their abuser. Make no mistake a person that does not love their child IS an abuser. Abusers are bad people and have no worth. Some people get brainwashed by bad, mean people. If you are a good person then you are fully entitled to have a wonderful sense of self. You have nothing to lose but those illusions…

As you focus on these words, you can know a part of you counts, and another part of you know what counts. Can you recall a time you were lightly entranced and daydreaming? Sometimes I'm talking to you, and sometimes I'm talking to YOU. As you continue to read these words imagine a bolt of lightning strikes the top of your head, zapping away all that old, mean brainwashing. You could imagine taking out your brain and cleaning it. You wash away all those mean ideas and plop that brain back in place - renewed. See the real you over there in your mind's eye, make the scene colourful, bright, attractive. See a swirling cloud that is the colour that represents *unconditional love* to you. Let it engulf that you. Filling every cell of your mind-body-spirit with total acceptance and love. See that feeling fill that loving you up. See the look on that you who is filled with a healthy sense of self-worth. You are a good person. You just know it and feel it. When you're ready…step or float into that new, real you. You are filled with self accepting thoughts and it feels wonderful. Bathe in that blissful feeling. Feel how good that feels. Lock these thing in. Keep them permanently as a gift to yourself. Read this section again two more times if it helps. Another dreaming part of you can complete this process whilst you doze. A willing unconscious can do many healing things at night. Under the stars.

YOU ARE GOING TO DIE!

I'm afraid the root cause of most confidence-sapping fear is a misplaced fear of death. Some people with phobias imagine they will become so scared they might die of a heart attack. They start to fear the sensations of fear. That's no fun. It is a fact to be faced that we are all going to end up pushing up the daisies. If you're an Atheist, well you shouldn't worry because for you nothing happens after death. Chill. Perhaps you are 'religious' and believe in an afterlife. Well, if you do, if you've been good, you'll go somewhere nice. What people are really afraid of is dying violently, painfully, and too young. If you're 110 when you go, that's not a bad innings. If you are in your teens you want to live a long life. By brother's friend raced his motorbike at an outrageously fast speed down one of the steepest slopes in the Surrey Hills. He came off his bike and...well, it was messy. Dead at 17, having done nothing. His last act, one of unthinking stupidity.

Don't want death, don't hasten it's eventuality: a good fear would be a fear of dying when you haven't finished what you're supposed to do here...

MEDIA: THE CONFIDENCE SAPPING MONSTER.

The media wants to sap all the joy out of your life. Look around you. See many happy shiny people laughing? The media exists to make you fearful and miserable. They exist to make you feel bad about yourself - they like to point out how morally superior to you they are without any evidence to prove such claims. THEIR JOB IS TO BRAINWASH YOU!!! They are staffed by an interchangeable private little club. And they really don't care for the general public riff raff at all. Terrorists! Murder! Drugs! Baby killers! Rape! Crime! A daily diet of fear, in a fearful society conjured out of thin air by the media. You should be careful what you let into your brain, for the mind has no firewall. Face facts, but don't let someone, who doesn't even care a damn for you and your family and friends, for your neighbourhood or country tell you what 'reality' is. It is a fact that the media industrial complex is rife with psychopaths. Make of that what you will.

CONFIDENCE AND 'SUCCESS'.

There is nothing quite like the thrill of success. It's a special, intoxicating feeling. **_Confident people do not fear competition._** We succeed at things every day. You succeeded in brushing your teeth. Eating something. Combing your hair, or at least making it presentable. You do some things very well. Is or are their 'secrets' to success? Yes...

1. Set your goal (we'll talk about this more in the next section).
2. Take steps to achieve goal.
3. Goal is achieved. Move on to the next goal.

A man came to see me and said he wanted to be 'successful'. I said, "What do you mean by 'successful?" he replied that he wanted to have lots of money. For him lots of money = success. Certainly having money is dandy. What do you mean by 'success'? Can you make a mental note of what success is for you? Can you write or type it down? How will you know when you have attained it? What specifically will have changed for you?

Success is often linked to 'ambition' - the origin of this word meant 'to go'. Often to go around and gain glory, votes, 'honour'. What are you ambitious to go around and do? How do you want to change your life for the better? Who do you want in your life? What resources, inner and outer will help you achieve personally meaningful things? You will need a plan. there's nothing wrong with planning, as long as **you** are doing it. Let no one else order your dreams. If you like, visualise now all the things you'd like to do in this life....take you time...let your mind wander...this isn't pipe dreaming...this is success rehearsal...being ever mindful of your realistic progress...and changing certain things...that need to be changed...doing that which must be done...as you find yourself succeeding more often. Because that's what confident people do. *You are a winner!*

GOAL SETTING.

Now, you need to choose _worthy goals_. Yes, they should benefit you, but they mustn't harm good people. If your goal is knowledge, then you must find the right source. If your goal is excellence, then you must learn from those who excel. If you goal is 'more money' then do things that bring in more money. If you want to swim you'll need some water...If you could only succeed, what goals do you really want to accomplish in this life? Go on a little thinking gumble...or right them all down. How much control over the goal achievement process do you have? The closer it is to 100%, the more likely it is to happen. Goals that require the involvement of others require some kind of persuasion. So remember to persuade ethically. Make sure the people you aim to make alliances with are fair-minded. A real person's word is their bond. So it is with honourable people at least. If you go for something with all your heart and soul you may surprise yourself. Never do anything worthwhile by halves. Commit!

KEEP LEARNING.

Unfortunately a large number of people have a fucking slow learning curve. They can't see the shit from the shinola. By the time they're in the shit, it's too late to avoid treading in it. They're knee deep in shit, and sinking fast. Then they can't work out how they got there. **_This is why you need to pay close attention to that which is actually going on around you._** Not what you wish or imagine or believe. You are entitled to believe what you want, but that don't make it so. Most people assume too much without enough facts. Often without any. The grapevine is fine for wine, lousy for a map.

I was once on holiday in Hastings on the south-east coast of England. As I and two others walked back from a session at a series of pubs, we staggered back to our hut on the cliff summit high above. To get where we were going we had to pass through some gorse scrub. As we walked and laughed a bright trailing object about the size of a soccer ball flew over our heads and zoomed off into the distance. "Did you see that!? What the fuck was that?!" It was clearly some kind of thing composed of light, someone replied seriously, "It was a seagull. It must have been a seagull." If that was a seagull on fire it wouldn't have looked like that. Even if a flying dick lands on someone's nose and farts in their face, some people just can't face the truth. Confident people can. There are more things in heaven and earth Horatio…speed up your learning curve or repent at leisure.

Never stop learning, there's always so much more to learn…I had an old man who couldn't read tell me it was 'too late' to learn. I told him *in hypnosis* that it's never too late to learn what you want and need, now…

CREATING YOUR LIFE'S WORK.

What is a 'life's work'? Well part of the purpose of being human is to go through the natural human life cycle. You grow up, learn shit, get a job or jobs, have some kids, get old and...your life's work is the sum total of the total unfolding of you in the material world. Your life's work may be to study x, to do y, to boldly go... somewhere or other. We are all on unique paths. Sometimes they intersect briefly, with meaning. With others there are clashes. Just not on the same wavelength. There are dark, failed souls out there too, you must be on guard against them. Your life's work will occur when you make it happen. But I suggest you have a life's work. It creates a story line on which to hang the tapestry of your life. Make sure it's 100% what you want to devote yourself to.

GETTING YOUR HUMAN NEEDS MET.

For some logic defying reason, humans don't think they need to do certain things. Plants have needs - they need water and sunlight. If they don't have these two things they die. Humans need good food without pesticides on them. Good food means 'organic' food. Organic plants are filled with vitamins and minerals. And probably lots of other things a nutritionist could tell you about. When you eat right you might not even need those vitamin pills. Did you know that most obese people are malnourished? Most overweight people are addicted to highly sugary foods. Certainly they eat too many bad carbs. I once had a rather officious spinster teacher come to see me. She wanted help with weight loss. I asked her to outline her usual 'diet' for me. She ate tons of cakes and sweets every day. I said, "You are not eating food. A cake is not food. It has no nutrition in it." Now, this is an exaggeration, but it's close to the truth. If you eat mainly cakes - you'll be doing great for carbs and sugars. Where is the protein? Where are all those lovely vegetables with natural magic goodness in? Anxious people often have bad diets. I would get my 'depression' clients to imagine buying healthy food from the grocery store/super market. I would get them to imagine making lovely meals for themselves. I'd get them to notice how all that nutrient packed food made them feel so much better.

There is a great little slogan I learnt from a natural bodybuilder - "Eat the rainbow!" I don't think he invented it, but it refers to the idea of eating vegetables with all the colours you can imagine. Purple, orange, green, white, bright red, you name it. The quality of meat you eat is highly important - factory farmed animals are so pumped full of junk you can't imagine, until you research it. Go 100% organic. "It costs too much!" Nope - it costs too much if you don't. I have found that by shopping around on online organic stores and doing price comparison purchases I can substantially cut my food bills per week. Whatever you do, never eat a 'Frankenfood'. We don't need genetically modified crops. Nature has been taking care of us for ages. It knows more about what we need than we do. Organic food also tastes of something. When you first go organic you'll start noticing that real vegetables are plump, juicy and uniquely tasty. The meat can't be beat. If you want confidence for life - go as close to 100% organic as possible. If you treat yourself with some junk every now and again, that's fine, don't sweat it. But, the core of your food intake must be organic. If you genuinely can't afford organic yet, find the best quality produce you can. The quality of your diet is intimately linked to a healthy, functioning, germ busting immune system. Your immune system can kick the arse/ass of anything if you feed it right.

Carb myth: carbs aren't bad for you - you need the energy, for your body and importantly for your brain to function; brain fuel is sugar. Bread is a staple - just eat good quality bread. Fat isn't bad for you, you need it, fat is where the flavour is stored in meat. You need salt: ignore the salt Nazis, they all look ill anyway. Another tip - never take health care advice from someone who looks like crap. Good food is natural medicine and preventative medicine. Eat eggs, creamy butter, steaks, the lot! When you eat more nutrition filled organic food you'll crave less snacks. Most people without emotional problems eat snacks because they are malnourished; with organic food that won't be a problem. Your food bills will go down. Now let's talk about exercise.

You must exercise. Even if your diet is just okay - a regular exercise routine, I'll define this soon, is the stress buster par excellence. Exercise makes you feel good without drugs. Your mind and body, once looked after properly will produce all the natural uppers and downers you need. You sex life will improve, you'll look more attractive. When you feel more attractive, you'll feel much more confident. Although attractiveness is about 90% attitude, but that's another story. Regular exercise flushes out stress.

Let me explain. When you feel fearful, stressed, anxious, angry, worried, frazzled etc., let's just say you've had one of *those* days, exercise is your magic, 100 natural and free silver bullet to feel good again. Exercise isn't a maybe, it's a must. You need to exercise. At least 3-4 days a week. You are not just a head on a stick. Appreciate your body. It's amazing. In many ways it is the 'subconscious'. It has a wisdom to fight disease. It extracts goodness from food. It gives you hunches - that gut feeling; listen to it. Your body is your survival suit on earth. It's you in physical form. Look after it. Care for it. Exercise. Exercise. Exercise.

When we become stressed our body releases chemicals to prepare us to face the danger. Imagined dangers and a perceived attack on our ego can trigger this stress response. We'll get to that. Allostatic load is the technical term for the wear and tear on mind and body from chronic stress. Exercise reduces allostatic load, and gets rid of it. Zebras that have just been chased by lions 'shudder out' allostatic load. But we aren't zebras, we are humans. Humans exercise to get rid of stress. As long as you don't abuse alcohol that can help with temporary stress relief, but you can't reach for the booze in the middle of the day if someone drives their car dangerously close to yours. Go for a walk, one that makes you sweat slightly, jog, hit the gym, or dig out those rusting, cobwebbed weights at home. Go for a swim. Watch that old Cindy Crawford exercise video. Play a sport. Go dancing. Whatever takes your fancy. You must break out into a light sweat for it to work.

A word on gyms. If is quite easy and cheap to make an effective home gym if you have the space. I personally can't stand UK gyms. Full of posers. And I used to be a bodybuilder! You must find the exercise routine that's right for you. Before I work out I stretch, some people don't have to. We're all different. Gaining confidence is about finding out what is right for you. As you try out differing activities that make you feel good naturally, and de-stress you - you'll be learning about you. Why do we learn? To increase our level of control. That's why other people recommending what exercise you need to do is dumb. If you enjoy golf and you feel better after playing it - do that. Experiment, design your own exercise routine, read books, get tips off YouTube, anything. Become your own expert on what exercise de-stresses you.

<u>DRUGS!</u> The 'recreational' use of drugs is one of the most awful signs of a decaying society. We are living through a new 'Opium War'. The West is being destroyed by drugs by design. If you are using so-called recreational drugs or potentially dangerous psycho-active substances of any kind you'll never you'll never be fully confident. How could you be when you are damaging your health? Anything that degrades your body and mind will only rob you of confidence and self-respect. Pornography is a drug, a mild one, but a drug nonetheless. The widespread use of cocaine was the most prevalent major drug addiction problem I was presented with as a therapist. Cocaine is funny, it's not physically addictive, but it can be psychologically addictive. All social classes in England do it. I have been waiting in a line in a pub to use the toilet and all around me were young men waiting to snort shit up their noses. Cocaine use is normalised, almost part of some people's lifestyle. Cocaine is the classic drug of Generation Narcissist. Why? Cocaine makes totally irrelevant people feel they are important. This is why both psychopaths and people with low self-worth love it.

Drugs don't improve self-worth - they rob you of it. Your mind produces all the uppers and downers you need, naturally, when you live a healthy lifestyle. Drink alcohol sensibly. I know of 70 year old men who drink like sailors on shore leave. They collapse and crack their head on the pavement and end up with bleeding on the brain. Booze can calm you down, at first, but it also lowers your inhibitions and stops you from controlling your emotions. Excess booze makes you more nervous not less.

To conclude: confident people can enjoy moderate alcohol, but cut out all psycho-reactive drugs now. That includes cigarettes. Nicotine cigarettes are one of the most insidious forms of addiction ever created. If you can't stop using drugs yourself - get help. You can read my book on addiction: **Hypnotically Deprogramming Addiction**, but you might need a skilled therapist.

Privacy. Yes, in our heavily monitored world, I'm afraid you need your own space. We have this need even in childhood. By about age 10 we need time to go off and do our own thing for a bit. Parents worry that little Jonny hits his teens and goes off into his room a lot. He needs to. It's normal. If you don't get enough privacy you can develop anxiety problems. Some people need more privacy than others. Respect this.

Companionship. People need people. We need to connect to some people, not on a superficial level, but on a deep level. Do you have at least one person in your life that you feel a deep connection to? No? Go and make new friends.

People think its great when you have lots of friends: are they really friends or just acquaintances? The latter can be good fun, you can have a chat etc., but ultimately there's no real connection. You may go through phases where you have more friends than at other times. You can go off people. Grow to like new ones. I have dumped ex-friends, just the same as I've dumped ex-girlfriends. You outgrow people. As you become more confident you'll begin to notice that you'll give off an aura that attracts people to you: you'll have your shit together. Paradoxically you'll also become pickier. You'll suss out the fair-weather friends from your core lifelong friends; the latter become family.

There is a wonderful Charlie Brown cartoon that always stuck with me. Charlie Brown is at summer camp and he's writing a letter to his parents. He writes about a boy he has met and they have struck up a friendship. In parallel storytelling panels we see the boy is writing the same letter to his parents. They both end their letters in unison saying,"*...He will make a great temporary friend."*

<u>Meaningful work.</u> My dad was a trade unionist. He had a book called, 'Useful work versus useless toil.' The author wrote about the difference between meaningful work vs doing a job you hate to survive. Now we all have to work. As an adult most of your day will be spent involved in doing a job of some kind. You have to eat, pay the bills, have a roof over your head, and buy clothes etc. You want that place in the 'Burbs! Ultimately you want a job that gives you financially security and independence. When you have those two things you'll have confidence. But, if you work in a job that is soul destroying you will rapidly lose self-confidence. Let me explain, you gotta do what you gotta do. When you get your first job you have to do crappy jobs. You don't have any skills to sell. I cleaned tables and served food. You have nothing anyone else wants. Anyone can clean, work in a shop, serve food, drinks etc. It's low skilled work. There is nothing wrong with doing any job as long as you get something out of it.

Some people lack the guts to go after what they really want. This reminds me of Billy Joel's song 'James'. A song about a man who does a job to please everyone else but himself. And he is obviously miserable. Your life is your life: as the song says - 'Do what's good for you, or you're not good for anybody...'

This all has to do with confidence. A confident person just knows their calling. They know what they are here to do. It might be several things. But something inside them, their natural inclination and talents lead them to their destiny. I believe from very early in life we know our destiny. What we are meant to do. It sings out to us from within. Most are too afraid and turn from the call. A confident person never does this. No matter what the odds or obstacles. Be who you were meant to be. Do what you gotta do in the meantime: but make that dream come true. That's what 'reaching your potential means'; it mean doing what you were meant to do. Be responsible, work to make money to take care of yourself, but learn what you gotta learn, have the experiences you need to experience, and **live the dream**.

At some point we reach 'the turning point', actually there are several, many. It's that point when we know if we do something our life will never be the same again. It takes guts, but when we go through that doorway…On boy!

<u>*Connection to something bigger than you.*</u> Somehow in some bizarre almost telepathic way, we all all connected to one another. ***One of the most powerful transformative forces is a truly original thought.*** You see, most people are parrots. They just repeat ideas they've been programmed with. A truly confident, independent-minded person thinks original thoughts. They just pop into your head, when it works correctly. When you think it, it goes out there. Thinking an original thought is contagious. Other people soon start thinking along similar lines. How it gets out there? I have no idea, but it does. And trust me, the powers that be know all about it. Why do you think powerful groups spend so much time and energy programming people? So they can be original? No, so that they are predictable and controllable.

When we feel a connection to someone, something, some group it gives us a joyful sense of meaning, purpose and enrichment. A confident person is an individual yes, strongly individualistic, but we need to connect with, be with certain others. It is enjoyable to share experiences with those we care for, who share our values. We may even feel this sense of connectedness simply by listening to the same radio show. Sports fans feel it at the stadium: we all feel a powerful urge to communion.

Respect your ancestors: don't piss on their memory. They fought, loved, died, grieved, felt joy, were conquered, freed themselves, did great and petty things, were cruel and kind, had profound experiences, you are them bottled up in one body. You are the wisdom of your ancestors. You are descended from millennia of survivors. Never forget that, never disrespect their life's struggle. You owe them.

This natural communion urge is exploited: especially by leftists. They create artificial communes to replace the natural ones they destroyed. It's a form of social drug addiction. But we truly find communion in the family, extended family, the region we live in, tribe, nation, ethnicity, race, religion, creed, clan, club of shared interests, consumer gang (for example YouTubers who are into pop culture etc.) We find communion when we connect with people on the same wavelength. The 'Asylum-System' tries to make you feel alienated and lonely. That you are eccentric, that you should just conform. Actually most people secretly think like you. Confident people never conform.

A cause. There is nothing more motivating in this world that a cause. In his 'An Actor Prepares', the acting teacher Stanislavski posited the idea that a character in a play had all the actions that they carried out 'hung' on something he called 'the super objective'. What is *your* super-objective? Do you have a grand master plan you want to achieve? Are their certain things that you seem to be naturally drawn toward? Our natural talents and abilities often guide us toward finding our personal super-purpose. The overriding principle that governs the overall chain of our actions. A human without a purpose is like a car without fuel. A kite without the wind. Super-objectives pull you forward in life. There is nothing more soul-destroying than just existing. Just doin' the 9 to 5 grind, watching TV all the time, and eating…shit. You need to liven yourself up darling. You need, if you haven't got one yet - a cause. Go find your cause. It is not for me or anyone to tell you your cause. You will find it. Or, perhaps, it will find you.

Connection to your life's purpose. Related to this is the idea of your life having a unique purpose. Like Superman, you are here for some special reason. I don't know what that is, you do. Deep inside you were probably born knowing it, or it developed in you as you observed the world. It need not be grand. But it can be. People are trained to think that 'special' people achieve certain things. No, no one is born out of a special or better vagina than anybody else.

Shakespeare wrote: "There's a divinity (fate) that shapes our ends, rough hew them how we will." You can't change the family you were born into, the race, the ethnicity, the eye colour, the spirit of the times that exists as you enter this beautiful, crazy, at times evil, weird world. But no matter what hand fate dealt you, play it well my friend. For they are yours and yours alone. John Lennon said that life is what happens when you're making other plans. That said, we must carve out own fate if we are not be be mere automatons of powerful corrupt people, the programmers - that want you to act as they say. The weak and jealous that would drag you down to their degraded level. You must trust your own judgement. You must follow you own calling. If we are spirits descended for a purpose, as I know we are, then our stay here, brief though it is, has inherently therefore the deepest and most profound of meanings. Make yours count: make your mark on this world. In some way make it a better place. If you haven't already - find your life's purpose: shape YOUR future. You've got one life. Live it fully, without fear. There is no evil that cannot be faced if you are bold. You are a doer!

<u>**Love of truth.**</u> Lies are the propulsion fuel of madness. I will write more on this in a separate section later: here, I will say this. You cannot be confident if you are not a truth seeker. **Truth is THE foundation of confidence.** No one built a castle with marshmallow or wispy clouds. You need the rock of truth. When you engage with truth, every second of every hour of the waking day, your confidence will reach heights you cannot now possibly imagine.

<u>**Appreciation of beauty.**</u> One of the defining aspects of Western Christian Civilisation was beauty. Marxism hated this beauty. You see this in the urinal as 'art' (Marcel Duchamp 1917 - the year of the Bolshevik Revolution). The uglification of the arts, human relationships, political covenants etc. has degraded humans over the last 100 plus years in unimaginably horrible ways. In Britain this process really took off under the creature formerly known as

'Tony Blair'. Blair's government entirely destroyed the arts in Britain. It destroyed the music industry entirely. Britain is a country that grows uglier, dirtier and more destitute by the day. You only need look at the disgraceful shambles that is Gatwick Airport, the first thing that a foreign visitor sees on entering England, to realise that collectively Britain is a fat, ugly slob with no self-respect.

It is a must to develop an appreciation of true beauty. This is a personal things. I cannot advise you on it other than to say that beauty creates confidence. The expression and pursuit of beauty in all its forms: you must seek this. Confidence grows amongst beauty. Not amongst urinals, the bestial, the venal, and the pathetic. There is a natural nobility found in confidence. A dignity. If you do not behave in a naturally dignified way, as even the poorest once used to do, how can you consider yourself truly confident? A confident person has standards. There is more poetry in the intricacies of a leaf than...

Creativity. Confident people are creative. Anyone can destroy something: destruction is easy. Armies kill and smash. All that corrupt people do is destroy. *It is their very reason for existence.* A confident person is the type of person that picks up the pieces and builds something new. Creativity is that most human of endeavours: above all else it is probably our capacity to create that separates us most from the animals. That and the fact we don't lick our genitals in public. Well, I don't.

Building anything is creative, a house, a snow man. Drawing, building a business. Writing a letter. Creativity fully engages all of us. The unconscious provides the flow of ideas and inspiration, the conscious is that practical fellow that makes it all happen with diligence and hard work. Once the initial creative phase ends, the phase of prolonged, sustained effort takes place. This is when you make the idea a reality: this can take time. Five minutes or years. Confident people have the energy to sustain such efforts, knowing that the end result makes it all worthwhile. By doing we learn. If one creative effort is unsuccessful, you try another. That's the way the cookie crumbles.

Human art, wonderful as it can be, is nothing compared to the creativity all around us in nature. This is good because no matter how talented we are, this fact keeps our feet on the ground. But we all have that little bit of creativity inside us. Creativity doesn't have to be expressed artistically - sportsmen and women are capable of amazing feats of physical creativity. A meal is a creative act if you take the time to make something of it. All master craftsmen get better over time. Practise makes perfect. Do the best you can, and accept that. "The next one will be better!" as the infamously bad director Ed Wood said.

What are you going to create now that you are unearthing the birthright of your restored confidence? Confident people create…the rest is up to you.

Being fascinated by what you do. Nothing in this world produces a natural, pleasant flow state better than being totally absorbed in what you do. When what we do is connected to why we are here, these flow states become very intense indeed. The world disappears when we are immersed in processes that have deep meaning for us. This may be learning from a book. It may be our job. It may be a challenge. It could be an absorbing conversation with someone truly interesting. Flow states are natural waking trance states that make us feel really good. With your new confidence, what new things, or old things reconnected to are you going to allow yourself to fully experience? Reorganisations can and do occur. And you can, can you not? That's right, didn't you? Things just need to shift in subtle ways, outside of awareness, that allow the new-old ways to shine…

Sunshine and fresh air are free. Look, to stay healthy you can just go outside and get some fresh air and sunshine; you need to, even in winter. The sun gives you lots of nice vitamin D - a super vitamin that also helps keep your immune system strong. Contrary to what you may have heard fresh air IS inherently good for you.

Some people, I had several clients like this, stay inside during winter time. They hibernate like an old bear. You need to get out, even if it's cold. I had a man who would buy some kind of artificial light because he got a made up thing called 'SAD'. He simply needed to go out more and get more sunshine on him. Fresh air and sufficient sun will make you feel more confident. I guarantee it. Don't get burnt.

There is a full and comprehensive list List of human needs in the appendix to my third book **Powerful Hypnosis**.

MOST PEOPLE ARE PREDICTABLE COWARDS - RELAX.

Lot's of people who 'lack confidence' imagine they live in a world of people who are vastly more confident, talented, intelligent, brave etc., etc. than themselves. Nothing is farther from the truth. Most people are conformists. Most people are abject cowards. Most people are either so dumbed down or so badly 'educated' that you shouldn't even worry about them in terms of competition.

It is a fact that most people do what they are told by almost anyone. No mater how low their moral character. Most people on this planet are happy to obey under any circumstances. Most people totally lack the guts to go for what they truly want in life and end up living 10th rate lives. Most people are both predictable and boring. Most people do the same repetitive, boring things over and over again. They eat the same food. Go to the same places at the same times like robots, or those little clockwork figures on Swiss clocks. Most people don't think, they repeat what they heard on TV or in the newspapers. You know that people are repeaters when they start a sentence like this: "They say..." Who are THEY exactly? People are trained to be predictable. Predictable people are controllable. If you want real confidence, do not be predictable. If you want real confidence become an interesting person who thinks interesting things and does interesting things. Be brave and ambitious. No matter what the circumstances, people who are genuinely confident build the kind of life they want regardless. *FUCK THE SYSTEM*. The system exists for parasites who live off of the productive.

If someone is a snob and looks down on you, you should thank your lucky stars, you have encountered a fool who underestimates you and your abilities. Snobs think in fixed ways which makes them predictable, like any other kind of small-minded bigot.

A confident person rejoices when others put obstacles in their way. What challenge is worth achieving if it's easy? The fact is unconfident people assume that others have a great many superior abilities which in fact they don't. Confident people can view themselves and others objectively. You need to *still your mind* and relax. Focus on what you want and then take steps it make it happen. As long as you are reasonably intelligent you'll do fine. You can become more and more intelligent. Intelligence is like a muscle.

STATUS AND CONFIDENCE.

I first learnt about 'status' when I was studying acting; it was something I had barely considered beforehand. If you take a king in a play and compare him to his jester, the king is higher status. The king sits calmly in his throne, when he speaks others listen. He only rises if he has to. He expects people to follow his commands. He does not plead with them. His posture is straight. You get the idea. Now the jester has to please the king. He has to make him laugh or he's out of a job. He jumps around, generally makes a fool of himself, and is anxious for applause. He juggles, he blows fire just to get attention. He expends much more energy than the king.

There are a series of behaviours that denote a low status character, you will never find them in a truly confident person. Low status persons have difficulty maintaining comfortable eye contact. Their shoulders hunch, the head is lowered in some way. Their feet can even turn inward. They clench or fidget with their hands. They speak too fast. They do not belly laugh but titter nervously. If they smile, it is a strained smile. Their forehead is wrinkled. They seek to hide, and may shorten their height even if tall, almost as though bowing to other people. They give off an apologetic air, they seem sorry to exist or to bother you at all. When they try to start a topic of conversation others speak over them. Do I need to go on?

Now, I don't want you to go around like a king. But, its time you started to carry yourself with respect. If you act as though *you respect yourself,* others will treat you with respect. You don't need to be angry, forceful, aggressive, 'assertive' etc. just start acting as if you matter: because you do. However I'd rather you acted like a king or queen than a fool. A lot of people in this world act like a nobody, be a somebody. You are actually a somebody you know.

TRAUMA AND CONFIDENCE.

Now, although I expect most readers to get something from this book, those who have experienced trauma, acute, chronic, extreme etc. may need to seek professional help. In my book **Hypnotically Annihilating Anxiety** I give fully details for how a hypnotherapist etc. can detraumatise someone; actually it's easy - you just use my How to Detraumatise Anyone script. I suggest you let a pro guide you through it. They may have their own tricks. But, if you've experienced trauma and nothing in this book works get professionally detraumatised. Trauma creates an energy. That needs to be transformed into its opposite: confidence. However, whoever you are, I bet you get something from this...

THINK LIKE A <u>REAL</u> AMERICAN.

I added this little section because I think most REAL Americans are CAN DO people. This is the complete opposite of British people who are can't do people. Confident people think like Americans. Americans are also more egalitarian than Europeans. They take you as they find you. My friend is half-American so I know. |They make very good teachers because they just get on with the job, and always know more than anyone else about the subject matter at hand. I have always found Americans to be more professional at their jobs. They go the extra mile. They think outside the box. They are more open to new, effective ideas. They are more generous than Europeans; they're also much more gracious. They aim to be the best; if they're teaching you, they want you to be the best you can be. This is something very alien to the haughty British, white, middle class, mediocrity loser, amateur mindset that is so pervasive that it actually drags the entire UK down with it.

If you want to do anything remotely unique: think like an American, even if you aren't one. You might even develop that confident charm that Americans have.

PHYSICAL HEALTH AND CONFIDENCE.

Do nothing that endangers your physical well-being: ever. If we are injured or ill we can lose confidence. If you are physically impaired or damaged, even disfigured for one reason or another you can lose confidence. But not to worry - confidence is an inner thing, not an outer thing. Any outer based tricks in this book affect the inner realm.

Exercise is good for its stress busting ability but its also a great way to maintain health. l people have hope. And he who has hope, has everything, as the Arabs say. As a confident person you must live a healthier lifestyle: don't be a saint. Have fun, but take care of yourself. If you are healthy your immune system works.

Men have a problem here: they are far less likely than women to seek help if they suspect a health problem. I knew a man who waited two years to get help for a leg pain. Don't wait two years for anything like that, it isn't macho to not face up to your problems. A double negative? Yeah, so what?

A word on hypochondria: it's bad for your health. Obsessing over being ill will make you ill. Anxiety over your health makes you more likely to catch something. You know the most important thing you can do to protect your health? Wash your hands after you take a shit. You ever seen men in a public toilet? Use the soap and water you dirty bastards.

FORMING A CONFIDENT GANG.

Now, it's far easier for a confident person to achieve goals if he or she has allies, like-minded people with the same goals and values. I suggest you *form a confident gang* of friends, relatives, colleagues etc. who work together. People need people. All of the greatest joys in life occur in relation to other people. Your little or big confidence gang will back you up in times of trouble. This is why people live in tribes, nations etc., to have a back up gang. You can be picked off one by one without a gang. Gangs give you protection. Gangs get things done more quickly. This is why some workers form unions - they get better terms and conditions. Sometimes it's impossible to achieve goals without other people, no matter how much of an individualist you are.

PLAN B: INSURANCE POLICIES.

Well we have 'insurance' if something goes wrong. Things can and do go wrong. You need to accept that as just being part of reality. This is one reason why we save money. Why we have pet insurance, health insurance. Some people are preppers. They don't look so crazy now, do they? Do you have preparations for a black out? What would you do if you lost your job? Do you need to get a will drawn up? I want you to come up with a series of plan Bs. "What would I do if…x, y, z occurs?" If you brainstorm, you'll come up with some contingencies for a rainy day. You can 'positive think' all you want; sometime shit happens. The question is are you prepared? Confident people are.

ABOUT WORRY.

The biggest thing that destroys confidence is worry. I'm going to teach you how to control worry. Worry is a little mind loop. You loop it over and over again. You can stop this "What if, what if, what if!?" process by noticing when you're doing it and saying "STOP!" in your mind and focusing attention on your surroundings.

Worrying is normal. Everyone does it a bit, when faced with a stressor. It's excessive, uncontrolled worry that's the problem. If you worry you create catastrophe scenarios in your head. If you see worrying pictures in your head drain all the colour out of them, make them black and white, make them tiny, and zoom them away into infinity. You don't have to do all this stuff for the rest of your life, it does help interrupt unhelpful patterns and habits until the confidence thing just kinda takes over. It will.

Write your worries down. Once they are there, out of that head on paper you can analyse them. You have made them objective. How many are there? Fewer than you thought? Turn them from worries into problems to be solved. ***Don't put problem solving off. Solve problems as and when they arise.*** Ask yourself: how likely is this worst case scenario likely to occur? Rate it's probability from 0 -100%. Most imagined fears that people have never materialise. If they do, you'll survive.

As the unconscious mind is so good at solving problems simply imagine writing your problem on a piece of paper. Put it in an imaginary bottle. Sling it behind you in your mind's eye. This sends a symbolic signal to the deep mind that you want that specific problem solved. Now get on with your life; forget about that. When it's ready, the unconscious will pop the solution/s into your mind.

Worry has the useful purpose of making you aware of potential dangers. I had a man who came to see me because he saw problems everywhere. He was an engineer, that was his job. To look out for problems on railway lines to prevent future accidents. Problem was he took his work home and couldn't stop. I suggested in hypnosis, whatever that is, that he compartmentalise that ability to appropriate times.

Panic can be stopped by demanding more fear. You just go into a situation that scared you and demand more fear. You taunt yourself and say, "Is that it!? More! The worst terror ever now!" and it goes. Your fear of fear makes fear worse. If you want to stop worry you worry more: if you are imagining the worst, you haven't gone far enough. Let your imagination go nuts! Imagine a scenario that is so bad, so ludicrous that it leads in some hilarious way to the annihilation of the entire universe. It should include nuclear war, and probably an alien invasion, and flying, machine gun toting great white sharks. If you're going to imagine crazy shit, at least make it fun. When you do: worry goes. Worrying is a misuse of the imagination. The imagination exists to make you generate solutions. And create new things. Calm down, let the surface of the water become still, it then reflects what is, without all those ripples, and use your IMAGI-NATION for what it was designed for.

You can get rid of some mild phobias by imagining the worst. Say you have a fear of vomiting. Imagine vomiting over people in a shopping centre/mall. Imagine uncontrollably vomiting over everyone, and being stuck like it forever. When you imagine the very thing you're phobic of until it becomes ludicrous it loses its hold. You are no longer a worrywart. You are confident, use your imagination the right way. You'll feel more confident, I promise.

Another thing to do to end worry is to keep your Jiminy Cricket and get rid of your Grima Wormtongue. People whose conscience is their guide have no need to worry. 'JC'? Same initials as...

DON'T BE A PEOPLE PLEASER.

Confident people break 'rules'. Fucking rules! Rules are for children. I once had a lady come to see me about a disfigurement that had occurred. But that wasn't the problem. She felt guilty about surviving a car crash in which others hadn't been so lucky. But that wasn't the problem. She was a people pleaser. This meant that she thought she had to do stuff for others to make them happy. This is a nice idea, but it generally leads to someone being treated like a door mat. We all need boundaries. We all have limits. You can't solve everyone else's problems. Often, when you try to help the 'innocent' they duck and you smash into a wall. Help people, but make sure you take care of your needs. This woman was so used to doing things for others, putting them first, that she didn't even have enough time to shit. I had to stop her feeling constipated all the time. When I freed her of the people pleaser addiction she exploded in honest fury at all the people who had exploited her kind heart. I had to help her calm down a bit. But sometimes it's good to get stuff off your chest.

A confident person can help others. But they are not 100% responsible for solving everyone else's problems. Sometimes the person you need to focus on is you. A confident person is not a people pleaser. Confident people are nobody's doormat. You can confidently say, "Sorry, not today, I'm doing...whatever..." Relationships are all about balance. You scratch my back. I'll scratch yours. If you're always scratching their back...?

Confident people aren't selfish, far from it, but you can't bend and twist yourself in order to become someone's idea of what and who you are – for their convenience. Life isn't a game of Twister. A confident person is firm but fair.

APPEARANCE AND CONFIDENCE.

Another thing I noticed about people who came to see me, the one's who were down in the dumps, was that they didn't take care of their appearance. They dressed shabbily. Their hair was unkempt. If you want to do one thing to aid your confidence - go buy a new outfit. I'm serious, get your hair done. If you don't want to splash the cash - just dress up a bit. Even if you're going to the shops/stores. People who lose their confidence stop caring. They think, "Oh I'm so blue, scared, a failure etc. Who cares how I look?" Well you should. Dress how you want, dress in the way that expresses your personality, but remember what ZZ Top said, "Every woman loves a sharp dressed man." Well, when a lady takes the time to make the best of herself: ditto!

Confident people are worth it: you are worth it. Go treat yourself. You should treat yourself now and again. Don't break the piggy bank...

CONFIDENT PEOPLE ARE HAPPIER.

When you are a very confident person you will *feel happy most of the time.* A fearful person cannot be happy. Fear trumps happiness. Confident people laugh more, see the funny side, look for ways to laugh even when things seem totally nuts, as people are saying a lot now, "The world seems to have gone mad." As indeed it has, by design. The ruling class of the world is at extreme odds with the citizenry. But every attempted absolutism that has ever existed always falls. They never last. You can feel confident and happier knowing that. People reach the enough is enough moment and get rid of tyrants. We are all going through a cleansing process, grim as things seem, on the other side will be a better today and tomorrow. You were born in historic times. No one will experience this again. You are here to witness the truth and to change reality by picking a side. If you pick the side of goodness, then you should feel very happy. If you chose poorly. I pity you.

There are so many things to be happy about. The people that you love, and that love and care for you. The beauty of nature. Great human achievements. The beauty of the blue sky is free. Good food. Fun. Games. No one can legislate away your sense of humour. People become happier when they take back control over their lives, happiness without freedom is impossible. How can a caged lion be happy, when he's meant to be roaming around the wilds of Africa? Confident people cede their personal power and responsibility over their life to no one. It's up to you. Be joyful, kind, cheerful and pleasant. Or as people used to say, "Don't let the bastards grind you down!" There is great joy in besting a worthless adversary.

YOU CAN'T MAKE UP A FAKE YOU.

It is better to be the real you and have but one true friend then pretend to be a character you invented because you want to be popular. You might call this 'performative confidence'. Outwardly confident, but inside? These types are easy to spot coz they act like dicks.

Being popular is one of the most overrated life goals there is. You know who's bothered about their popularity? Politicians. The planetary shit-heads. You see some person and think: "Oh look, they're so popular, everyone loves them. I wish I was just like them." For all you know they're secretly an axe-murderer. Why does it make you better if 5 more total fucking strangers like you? So what? What do you care? Some socially nervous people worry about every social encounter, even with someone at a shop/store. Relax - they don't give a fuck about you. You're just the billionth face that hour.

I knew a man who knew another man who fancied this particular woman. He found out what she liked and pretended he liked it to. You know what happened: she just got fucked by some other total loser. What a big old waste of time. If he had been his true self, if he even knew who that was, he would have at least kept his self-respect. Unless it's to preserve your life etc. don't perform/act in real life. You are fine just as you are. You don't have to be someone else's puppet. You can like what and who you like. You can hate what and who you want. Hate is normal. You damn well better hate some things. You don't have to be agreeing with people you disagree with. You can't escape *you*. It's about time you were confidently you. Know, there's a nasty version of this problem. It's called narcissism. More on this in a mo'. What I just talked about is the 'inferiority complex' version. Why would anyone feel inferior to anyone else? Just because someone imagines themselves superior doesn't mean you should jump in and join their delusion.

When people lack confidence they often end up as the 'sidekick'. They attach themselves to some dominant personality, like a little, distant planet rotating around the sun. They let the dominant personality become their guru. As they do this the unconfident person, who hasn't found themselves yet, gets to hide. You get to become someone's gimp. A flower grows up toward the sun. You don't need to be someone's poodle; someone you imagine has 'their shit' together. The person who has to get that together is you. If the world is a stage, it's about time you took the stage and played your part. There are no small parts.

CONFIDENCE AND HONESTY.

A confident person is basically an honest, trustworthy person. You are someone who faces people head on. Beware of the character who talks to you with his head turned at an angle. Villains are often in profile on stage.

Primarily a confident person is honest with themselves. This takes self-awareness and self examination. Not self-consciousness. Most people are not aware of what they are doing, they are incapable of self-reflection and therefore improvement. This reflection should not be harshly critical. It is just an honest assessment. We've all done things we regret. We have all done things we wouldn't like done to us. But, we can recognise what we did, and stop ourselves doing it again. Forgive yourself for being human. This moral corrective faculty seems unique to man, perhaps some more intelligent animals have it. I know cats that have more ethics than certain humans but...

An honest person says what they think: you have the right to your opinion, never justify yourself to anyone. You are entitled to be wrong. Honest people learn fast, because they see and admit when the mistake occurs. If you are honest you will have more energy and feel better about yourself. Lying makes the real you hide, as though you were ashamed of yourself. Are you? Why are you? Because you're not a supermodel? Or a top sport's star? The greatest X? None of those things matter. Stop comparing yourself unfavourably to others. Take the time now to acknowledge what you and you alone do really well....Think of a time you helped someone…and that help was appreciated…What are you good at?…What goals have you achieved that you are really proud of? What is unique about you?…What do your friends and family regularly compliment you about? Ponder this…

Honest people are relaxed with themselves. They are comfortable in their own skin. You're not perfect, and neither is anyone else. You are 100% human. You don't need to be anything else. You aren't here to impress anyone. You simply are. Don't expect from others what they are incapable of giving. Honest people are fun to be around, they're spontaneous, they have more energy. Lies waste energy. They shrink you, the energy of confident people focuses outward. Some people try to push your energy in, like a dog that's been beaten and cringes in the corner. Your energy goes outward to connect with the world, with reality, with other people. You impact the world in ways only you can. When you are gone, no one will do things as you did. Your impact is yours alone. It will never happen in another way through all eternity. There will only be one you. This is why every good person is special.

Confident people speak out when they wish, they can listen too. Confident people are a ray of sunshine in so many people's lives. Take the time now to remember a time when your honesty had some wonderful effect….perhaps you didn't expect it….Of course you should be wisely honest, not everyone deserves the revelation of the real you. There are times when honesty is not the best policy. You'll just knowingly know when it's appropriate. You were born honest, and then for some reason you thought you had to do things to please someone, to not be you but their imagined version of who you are not. Never conform to someone else's problems. No one who truly cares about another wants them to be what they're not. Honestly being you is your birthright. Embrace it. Mice are mice, no one wants them to be dogs. Lion's roar. The ocean swells and flows. The wind blows. Birds sing, Grass is green. Be who you really are…

A CONFIDENT PERSON FALLS IN LOVE WITH THE TRUTH.

This is the single most important factor in becoming confident. You cannot be confident, ultimately, if you do not love truth. Loving truth is the defining, make or break quantity in the confidence matrix. Truth is simply facts, that which is. You are there, interacting, in your own way with these words and ideas. That is a truth. Most people are trapped in a mind prison. This prison is a fake representation of reality. Reality is out there. There is no 'Matrix' out there controlling you. The only 'Matrix' that exists is the one that was placed in your mind, perhaps long ago. Almost everyone in human history has been brainwashed to believe in the ideas that a dominant minority at a given time wanted its servile class to have so as to better control them. That is a fact, whether the programmed you likes it or not.

Most people think their beliefs are facts. These are the worst and most pernicious beliefs that exist. Belief-factoids create assumptions. These assumptions make you believe in fairy stories and make decisions based on lies, myths, and half truths. Let's take the myths of the process known as World War 1. In this sociological event two competing imperial forces waged war against one another. Neither was morally superior in any way. The British Empire system won by getting the USA to win the war for them; without American intervention the British Empire would have been annihilated. Men from European heritage backgrounds were forced to fight against people who had never harmed them. If these men, who were Christians back then, refused to kill strangers for no good reason, they were shot. Have a good think about that if you are capable of doing so.

The world is no different now. People are just as willing to run out of metaphorical trenches into metaphorical gunfire and certain death as they were over 100 years ago. The majority of people are as dumb now, as they were then. That is a fact. If you don't like that fact that is your problem, it may well prove fatal to you at some point. Delusional beliefs can literally get you killed. One of the main causes of death on this planet must be fighting for a pointless or worthless cause.

Let's take an example of how most people process information: I say process information because most people cannot think. They have actually been conditioned to not like thinking very much, if at all. Say you have a belief:

"So and so is a nice man."

Let's just imagine you have this belief. Now what if the exact opposite is true.

"So and so is a very bad man."

Now, you are operating on the programmed-in fake reality that this so and so is a good person. Now, a truly brainwashed person will act thus when faced with a fact that refutes the delusion. Let's say that so and so kills his wife. It turns out he was raping and beating her whenever it took his fancy. Now, the truly brainwashed person will not accept the reality when confronted by it. A sane person will say:

"God! I was completely wrong about that person. He sure fooled me!"

This person will then create a little updated package in his or her mind that taught them something. That A was not B. They will learn something about being a bit too gullible and uncritical based on so little information. If I tell the brainwashed person that so and so did all those bad things to his wife and show him photographic evidence to prove it then I will simply get **the thousand yard stare**, as their eyes glaze over stupidly. They will them repeat their programming at you…

"I don't believe you. There's no proof of that etc."

This is when you know you're dealing with a zombie, of whom there are many. Most people are a mixture of brainwashed and sane. They are fact based in certain areas of information, and in others they are as immovable by contrary facts as is a big rock. You see **facts make you act!** Most people in our 'scientific age' believe they think scientifically. They don't. The difference true science made to the world is that it challenged and usurped power over written authority. Observation and experience were placed over ancient authorities. Whether these were of a religious or secular nature. Science 'said', you might believe that, but you can't prove it. If so and so was true it would lead to predictions that come true. For example, you may well believe that a ball will roll up a hill once dropped half way up the hill. However, I can assure you it will not. It will roll down that hill, unless something gets in its way, or it is met by an opposing force of some kind. This is because we now have a generalisation called, or known as 'gravity'. It existed before anyone believed in it or generalised about it.

Confident people think about things. Confident people trust their own experience. They trust their gut reactions. Confident people make decisions based on evidence. Words are not evidence. In the Ancient world authorities like Aristotle etc. made statement about reality that we would now simply laugh at. But for thousands of years the minds of educated men were swayed by garbage because Aristotle was regarded as a 'revered' (literally 'to stand in awe'!) personage. Never stand in awe of another human - ever. People like to forgo the responsibility of making their own decisions. They like to stay children their whole lives, letting other people make decisions for them. These people I would call confident babies, a baby is confident mummy and daddy will feed him. But when we grow up we have to feed and take care of ourselves.

You are responsible for the information you let into you head. You are responsible for developing a critical mind. You are responsible for your actions. In order to develop a truly powerful critical mind (the conscious mind) you must fall in love with the truth. You must examine the validity of your existing beliefs. You must let go of the comforting delusion that you know everything. You don't. I don't. No one does. You must seek truth: you must seek truth as though it were as vital as water to your well-being; because it is. ***It is not for me to tell you what truth is; that is a personal quest, which the confident person accepts. But, I offer you a warning. If you genuinely search truth you cannot go back. Ever. You will be changed permanently.*** But, you shouldn't worry, because you will only have 'transformed' into your true self. I will not help people be confident in possessing delusions.

As you bravely *go on your truth quest* you will not know your final destination. Truth quests can lead you to strange, and amazing places. You will have new experiences that you never expected. You will behave in more solid ways, as you make far better decisions than you have before. You will also be happier, even amongst great darkness. You will be calmer than you thought possible. Your mind will work properly; your analytical powers will skyrocket. You'll start noticing connections between things that you never suspected were in fact connected. You'll experience odd synchronicities that let you know you're on the right path.

You should practice sitting down or going for a walk and just thinking about a particular subject. What do you *really* know about it? Are you willing to read works by people you might disagree with? I can tell you something: truth is hidden in places you might least suspect it. You'll stumble across it after reading pages of boring waffle - then BOOM or POW, one sentence contains a truth and enriches you. This process doesn't end. It is the ultimate in 'self-improvement'. You see, you only have to observe children to know that ***EVERYONE THINKS DIFFERENTLY.*** This is natural: all children take words and use them in their own way. They prefer certain words and phrases, emphasise others. They start developing their own conceptual frameworks, as they see the world in their own way, through their experiences and they start to categorise it. And then, the 'controllers' start to step in and standardise children's 'thinking'; their brains are channelised to make them predictable and thus controllable.

Once you have broken free from your state induced programming trance you will start noticing the exact programs that other people have had installed in their heads. Then you will know how to steer, and even play games with them if you wish. Don't try to 'save' people. It's a good intention but some people are just fucking gone, and they ain't comin' back bar a miracle. Those who do not seek truth may accept some truths you tell them, partially. But they'll always warp it back to fit into their distorted programming. Jesus one said, "Let the dead bury their dead." The 'dead' are those who are not alive. That is, they have no truth or love of truth in them. They are the walking dead, of whom there are many. In the ancient mysteries, the 'dead' were the profane. The people who were not initiates into the mysteries. However, this was a lie because the initiates were the dead. It was an example of cult think. You might notice however that the walking dead are mysteriously attracted to you; after all zombies like brains.

Confident people love truth: if you haven't already, begin your search. It's yours alone. Do not fear the mob mind. Never let it sway you. Never follow the dead.

CONFIDENCE AND KINDNESS.

Are you a good person? "How good have you been?" someone once asked; that made me think! If you are basically a good person then relax, you are a person of worth. Most people are basically good. But there's more bad out there than most good people are willing to admit or face. A bad person wishes a good person harm: that's how you know them. A good person is kind. Not to everyone. You must be to yourself. Never put yourself down. Don't be too harsh over past mistakes. You can't change the past, you can learn from it, and make the future better.

Once upon a time in the West people had a religion. That religion said that being kind was the most important thing. The most human thing of all. Being kind demands discipline. It's easy to be an arse/asshole; that's why quite a few people enjoy being one. Babies need kindness as much as milk. Kindness makes everything more pleasant. This doesn't mean you have to go around loving everyone. People get kindness only if they deserve it. Being loving doesn't mean indiscriminately loving everyone, everything, every behaviour.

When people are kind we feel a special warmness inside. Someone took the time to care; so shines a good deed - in a weary world. Kindness is the gold of the human soul. If you're an Atheist, take that in a way that has meaning to you. If everyone is equally valuable, lovable, and deserving at birth, then what changed? It doesn't matter how much money you have. It doesn't matter how smart you are. How many books you read. Who your parents were or weren't. If you're famous or not. The most important thing is how good you are: caring is not something that needs training or schooling. It just requires that you be fully human. Confident people are kind…

DON'T TAKE ANY SHIT FROM ANYBODY.

Don't hang around people who don't respect you. One of the best ways to deal with a disrespectful person is simply to ignore them. If someone does something rude, do not react, do not engage positively with a person who is disrespectful until they show signs of submission and contrition. You must act like a high status person. A high status person is unaffected by low status people. Ignoring bad behaviour is a principle of animal training, and human training. Your face should be impassive. Remain relaxed. **_Do not use this principle on children; it is cruel._** Children feel unloved if they are ignored. We don't want to create any more unconfident people. Acting as if a rude person is tiresome or a bore, are also ways to go. You can look at your watch. You can simply leave the room, space etc. A rude person is almost always a person with delusions of grandeur - you must pop that imaginary bubble. **_Confident people expect respect._**

Having a full scale verbal sparing match is the last thing you want to do, but it is sometimes essential. Sometimes you must confront people. Sometimes you must have it out with people who are behaving badly. It can clear the air quite wonderfully at times. Do not engage in a verbal sparring match if you think you are dealing with a person who routinely resorts to violence. Many low IQ people think verbal sparring is the beginning of a fight. It is always better to use your wits. However sometimes you must be good at...

LIVING ACCORDING TO YOUR PRINCIPLES.

Principles. Can you recall a time you did something based entirely on your principles? You stood firm in the face of 'pressures', because it was the right thing to do. We've all done this. You must draw a line. You must have your own personal Rubicon. If you don't, slowly, but surely, you will start to erode your respect for yourself. If you don't respect yourself, you can be sure no one will. A person who lives according to their principles is a rock. The wind and rain may pelt down, but the storm clears and the rock remains. Mountains don't budge for anyone. People have been willing to die for their principles; not all of those were good people. But don't be stupidly stubborn. That has nothing to do with your principles.

Take some time now to ponder your principles…by considering them you can reaffirm what they are…who you are…what you value…what is right and wrong for you. A person without principles is a mercenary, a nobody, a prostitute. Confident people are none of those things.

You ever watch the Magnificent 7? About men who faced overwhelming odds to save a village from 'the baddies'. If you are truly confident - you gotta do the right thing. Don't worry about the people that don't do the right thing. Life has a funny way of catching up with the mercenary. Tick-tock…

ARROGANT PEOPLE ARE NOT CONFIDENT.

An arrogant person believes they are far more important than they are. They look down their nose at others. There are unfortunately many of these creatures. They are overbearing, insolent, assuming. They claim more than they deserve. They grasp for power. They like to tell others what to do. They claim more knowledge than they posses. They claim to have abilities and proficiencies they don't have. Most doctors I have met have been arrogant people. But, they're found amongst all races, classes, ages and professions. It is the smug sense of assumed superiority that makes them most loathsome. But, they are not confident. Often they come from 'privileged' backgrounds. I have watched such brats raised, first hand, they are verbally rewarded when they behave obnoxiously.

Confident people do not become arrogant. They're too sure of themselves. A confident person simply IS, and is grounded in reality. The arrogant pig is a creature who dwells in fairy stories and imagination. Like the troll, secure in his position under the bridge, until the moment the hero slays him. And reality dawns for the monster, a fraction too late.

STRENGTHEN THE WILL.

A confident person has a strong will. A confident person is determined to win/succeed etc., no matter what the scale of the challenge. In the face of setbacks and disappointments, which will occur, you must remain firm in your commitment to your goals and needs. Sometimes we have to make sacrifices for long-term gain.

The will is also essential for warding off addictive temptations. These include junk food, drugs (drugs destroy the will), porn, laziness etc. We live in societies that encourage an irresponsible, dissolute lifestyle. You must not succumb to it. This takes the active exertion of willpower. If you feel yourself wanting to indulge in any kind of wasteful lifestyle 'choices' imagine the negative consequences of doing so. Make the image big and colourful and painful.

The will directs the mind toward that which you really need. Though the will is strong it can easily be mugged by the emotions; this is why you must try to maintain a sense of calm. Calm minds work properly. Unless you are facing a charging Rhino, panic rarely solves anything other than making you unresourceful.

The will has nothing to do with dominating others; it has to do with self-discipline. Other-discipline is the worst kind, it makes individuals dependent and weak. Confident people have strong wills, they succeed, they conquer, they overcome: you are a confident person. Imagine yourself with strong willpower, getting done that which needs to be done. Will power is a quality found in people with *strength of character*. **You** have strength of character. You were born with it. Needed it. You have all you need within you. Reconnect to it. In...your...own....way. That's it.

NARCISSISTS ARE NOT CONFIDENT.

The narcissist or nazi-cyst is a vain form of arrogant person that has fallen in love with an imaginary self he's created. He actually fancies himself. He simply adores his fake self and believes everyone else must love 'it' as much as he does. But like the arrogant person, the nazi-cyst has feet of clay. His image is the reflection of a delusion. It is a mirage. **_Both arrogant and narcissistic people unconsciously model psychopathic behaviour._** A great many powerful and successful people are psychopaths. The higher up the greasy pole you go the more you find. As society encourages the emulation of the soulless ones, the weak-minded fall for the spellbinding qualities of those without conscience, and ape them. This is the danger of hypnotising someone to be 'confident'. They may have swallowed a lifetime of pro-psychopath propaganda through cultural hypnosis. Because they don't know who they are, and therefore can never be truly confident, the unconscious downloads the arrogant models it's seen who are 'successful' and manifests these in the conscious self's ongoing behavioural output. *BEWARE!*

A confident person is not fake, does not emulate the pompous, they are genuine, matter of fact, and not at all vain. They have a healthy ego. They have the confidence of things that ARE, not will-o-the-wisps that fly off with the slightest breeze.

DO YOU FEEL PHYSICALLY SAFE?

You can't really be confident unless you feel physically safe. You can beef up, learn self-defence. You can own a gun if you're American, but a dangerous environment is a risk to you. If you are able, get out of an environment that has too high a physical risk factor. There is such a thing as 'no go zones' on this planet; stay away from them.

Be aware of your surroundings: we live in increasingly dangerous times. A rising tide of neo-barbarism is sweeping the world and the West. Or what was the West. This will only worsen and you should not expect state operatives to come and help you, they'll be too busy trying to manage the coming crime explosion and carrying out their main duty which is to protect your rulers from you. Americans are much more aware of such things than are Europeans. The Europeans had better wise up fast. There is a wealth of information 'out there' on methods of improving your personal safety. Women I know are especially anxious about this. They should be. It is probably the most dangerous time to be a woman since the Dark Ages. Women especially need to be aware of physical risk in their environment. Avoid walking down dark alleyways at night. This is not the 1950s. If you see a gang of people and feel anxious about it, avoid them and take a different route. Any delusional beliefs you have about x, y, and z could lead you into harm. Confident people take measures to make sure they and their loved ones are safe. How you do this, in your own way, is up to you...

GOOD FEAR/BAD FEAR/ANGER.

Some people think that being confident means being fearless. Some people are fearless, which is fine, if you're not reckless. 'Bad' fear is imagined fear. That is, it is not based on any real danger, it exists in your mind only. Or it did, till now. People often feel imagined fear when they're put under some kind of stress or pressure. Propaganda is pressure applied to the mind. Pictures in a book are just that: pictures. No more mountains out of molehills. If you must use your imagination, use it to solve problems. Going for a walk, drive or bike ride, relaxing in the bath naturally allows the problem solving mind to wander and wonder its way to amazing solutions. They just pop in there. Relax knowing you have that ability. Never make a decision based on picture book fear. Do not allow others' words to make you afraid. Do you believe in spells?

Good fear protects you from real danger, you need it. Real fear gives you the energy to protect yourself. It allows you to pay attention, to take evasive or protective action, then it passes. So keep the real fear for things that are actually scary. But don't be ruled by fear, not even the real kind. Live with principle, even if there is fear. Fear not. Confident people find a way. Sometimes enduring is enough. But let's talk about anger…

Ah! The double-edged sword. It has its uses…don't let anger cripple you. Especially in stressful times. Yes, there are lots of bad, unjust, unfair things going on. If you cannot control that anger, you will grind yourself down and make yourself feel like crap. You can't fight everyone all the time. An enemy can use your anger to provoke you into fucking up. If you are swamped in rage you can't think.

Anger is often a response to frustration. X didn't happen. It is frustrating because what a problem sometimes needs is more time. You need patience to succeed. Anger can ruin relationships. Anger has its uses but don't let it possess you. The calm mind is the wise mind. Is a truly confident person permanently enraged? Where's your sense of humour? There is always 'karma'. A dish best served cold?

STOP BEING SO FUCKING NAIVE.

One of, if not THE biggest obstacle to your growing confidence, is being naive. Gullible people can never be confident. A lot of otherwise reasonable and intelligent people believe that rich and powerful people care about them. I am sorry to wake you up on this but, they couldn't give a fuck about you. It is best to have a very cynical, sceptical view on the powerful.

The lying psychopaths that run almost everything now couldn't care if you or your family lived or died, you are merely a means to an end to them. As a rule you should adopt a policy of having no respect for anyone in authority. Do not blindly do as they say or advice, think for yourself, do what you think is best. *By their deeds you will know them.* Never judge someone by what they say, but by what they do. Only trust long-trusted influencers. The time for unearned trust is over. Those times are gone.

For over half a century the corporate political class of the West have been sending all of the industrial capacity of the West to India and China. You have lost ancient liberties, hard fought for. Schools are seminaries of socialism. Men and women can't relate normally to one another. Broken homes, shattered lives, the new opium war, roads with potholes, ever rising taxes, wars that create refugees who are then imported, massive declines in Western birthrates, secular nihilistic Atheism replaces Christianity, poverty rising, neighbour turned against neighbour. Technology used to spy on you. Everything, every policy destructive. Home owners turned into renters. Why would you trust the criminals who did this to you? Are you sane? ***ARE - YOU - SANE?!***

Only trust people who deserve your trust. When you are 'betrayed' again, and again by people who were never on your side, the only person who conned you, was you. And beware the person who tells you what you want to hear, and then does something totally different. Once bitten, twice shy. Even an ant has a survival instinct.

MAKE BETTER DECISIONS.

Deep confidence comes from good information. This helps you make wise decisions. Wise decisions are the basis of confidence and true success. You can't be confident if you keep making fucking dumb decisions based on stupid assumptions. When making decisions of importance gather as much of the facts as you can, experiment; you do the research. Be your own journalist. Stop waiting for someone else to know what's best for you. Confident adults don't do that. Don't be mesmerised by 'experts'; trust me an expert is always selling something. Look out for the conflict of interests. The expert on what's best for you is not the Wizard of Oz, it's the person who stares back at you in the mirror. Confident people trust themselves.

But you, are here, and so you'll take steps from now on to get the best, most objective information you can. You'll compare and think. You may think some more. Then you'll act, wisely. And the better decisions you make will build better things - an unbreakable chain of confidence. If you make a mistake, then you'll dust yourself off and learn, really learn...

THE ATTITUDE OF A CONFIDENT PERSON 2.

Can you remember that time, in time, when you were deeply absorbed by something fascinating? A time you learnt some new things with ease. See what you saw, hear what you heard, feel that...now...What is 'hypnosis' anyway? Maybe it's this...

What colour is the colour of a confident person? What if all those *attitudes of confidence are inside* a cloud of confidence over there...There's a you over there...A you waiting for that confidence to take all that goodness inside the real you...See that new *confident you*, filled with all those confident ideas, and feeling, and good nutritious things as that colourful cloud of confidence seeps into every pore of your innermost being. *Feel that core confidence* - freed up, emerging from the depths of your soul. All that you were meant to be is in this...

When you're ready, step into that confidence...Step into that *confident you* over there - own it. Feel all that inside of you...Feel how it makes you think differently, feel differently, notice how you move, interact with others. What new insights do you have? What things have you've always wanted to do? Do them with all the commitment of all your heart and soul! I don't know how these changes will manifest, you do. It knows. It always did. As the two of you connect at a very deep level...you'll notice amazing things have already started, wasn't it? And a far deeper part of you is paying attention, nodding on the inside, it's about time, and in time, that willing part will carry out a process, during a restorative sleep, that will restore your birthright to YOU. And that's a nice thing to know, is it not?

DO NOT BE <u>THIS</u> PERSON!

There are two types of failure, amongst others: a failure of nerves, a failure of the imagination:

> 'The demonstration that no possible combination of known substances, known forms of machinery and known forms of force, can be united in a practical machine by which man shall fly long distances through the air, seems to the writer as complete as it is possible for the demonstration of any physical fact to be.'

Simon Newcomb. Astronomer.

Idiot.

CHEER UP: CONFIDENT PEOPLE ARE LUCKY!

I suppose 'luck' can be defined as a mixture of good fortune, things going your way more often than not, and an ability to make you own luck. Through your own efforts. Now, there is a lot of literature on the psychology of luck. I have to say, I think most of it is garbage. How do you scientifically prove 'luck'? Some boffins claim: "Luck is believing you're lucky." Yeah, right. I could hypnotise someone to believe they're lucky and they may well end up believing it, as hypnotised people often do. That don't make it so.

In my experience though, I would say confident people are luckier because they naturally demand more from life, from other people, from experiences than the unconfident. Unconfident people often end up with a spouse they settled for. They don't think they deserved better. I once had a woman come to see me who was working in a grocery store/supermarket job. She burst out crying and said, "I want a better job, but I'm too unconfident to leave." This is more common than perhaps many know. If you were unconfident until now, I bet you were selling yourself short. Lucky people, confident people demand more from life. They don't sit back and wait, they take action to improve things now. When faced with a problem they waste no time worrying, or procrastinating, they're too busying coming up with solutions and implementing them. I knew a young woman and whenever you came up with an idea she thought of at least 10 ways that you could make it happen. This is a most-deliciously anti-British mindset. The British are trained from birth to expect little out of life. That the 'world' is a NO kinda place. And if you believe that delusion - then you shall live it. He who lives by the delusion shall die by the delusion.

Confident people are lucky. They make YES things happen. As your confidence grows in the minutes, hours, days, weeks, months and years to come you'll notice that all these changes, these new learning feed back on each other: and that you become, somehow 'luckier'; whatever that means to you...

MAINTAINING CONFIDENCE:
Confidence for life.

In the immortal words of Seinfeld's Kramer, "Am I crazy? Or am I SO sane, I just blew your mind!" You may have been aware that this whole book is somewhat hypnotic...Now, your growing new confidence awaits the steps you take. You must take them, alone, but not lonely, and even though I am not with you physically. *I BELIEVE IN YOU MY FRIEND.* I am there cheering you on. And you are on a journey, the road goes ever onward. I don't know what will change for you. I do know one thing, it is an ancient wisdom... *write your own story...*

THE REST IS UP TO YOU...

Believe it or not, my next book is about WEREWOLVES! Patrons support is greatly appreciated! 4 Confidence boost visualisation bonuses follow...

APPENDIX 1: STEPPING INTO CONFIDENCE ETC.

The following requires no formal hypnosis: only light trance is required. To *enter light trance* you just need to visualise...

Pick an emotion/state you want more of: for argument's sake let's do confidence. With your eyes closed or open, whichever works best, and with enough space around you to walk about...

1. See/imagine a more confident you one step ahead of you. Make sure that image of a more confident you is super confident looking. Make it super bright and colourful! All the new attitudes and feelings are in there. When you're happy - step into that more confident you and *feel that confidence* soak deep within you.

2. Now, see another even more confident you another step or two ahead. Make sure he/she is really super confident, even more than the last step. When you're satisfied: step into that even *more confident* you etc. Feel this deep confidence flowing through every part of this even more confident you. Good...

3. Can you guess? Yes! See a third, even more super confident you. A you so confident that you glow with your colour of confidence! When you have that image just right, adjust it in any way to make it just right, step into that totally confident you. Everything you need is in here! Own this *deep confidence*. Let it seep into every pore. Let it go to the core of your being. That confidence just flows in and out, and all around you. That's it.

4. Repeat as desired. You can go two steps forward, then take one back etc. Then go three steps forward. Play: see what works for you.

APPENDIX 2: ANXIETY INTO CONFIDENCE.

The following requires no formal hypnosis: only light trance is required. To enter light trance you just need to visualise...

1. With eyes closed or open, whatever suits you best: imagine in vivid colour taking all that emotion you don't want: say anxiety etc. and holding it in a glowing ball of energy just in front of your solar plexus/chest area. Get a real sense of it. Imagine feeling it, moulding it with your hands...

2. Imagine a net, a hoop, a change portal, a basketball/netball hoop type thing that is glowing, powerful, and funky looking. Once you hurl that ball of anxiety etc. into that transformative object you will change that feeling into its opposite forever....Not now, but in a moment...

3. When you are ready bounce that anxiety up and down like a rubbery ball of something. After you've done that a few times: throw that ball of whatever into that portal! As you do notice a funky/wonderful explosion of colours shoots out of that 'hoop of change' etc. That change has occured.

4. Now, that energy ball is changed into your DEEP CONFIDENCE! With a will of its own it bounces back to you. Take it in your hands and feel its power! Now, place that feeling of turbo charged confidence inside of you, where it feels just right! That's it. Let that super-charged confidence go all through your mind and body and

out beyond you! Feel how good you feel: and keep that permanently locked in. Good.

5. Again, you can repeat this if it helps: say two times more. It's up to you.

APPENDIX 3: THE ROAR OF CONFIDENCE!

Light trance only required: eyes open or closed. Do what works.

1. Over there in your mind's eye see a 40 foot version of you filled with super confidence. Make it bright, colourful, attractive! That you can do anything within their abilities. They have strength of character and real power to affect the world positively. Notice how just looking up at that you makes you feel amazing!

2. See an animal that represents some emotion/state/feeling that you want more of. Hear that animal roar/cry out with a sound that represents your personal power! Feel how incredible that makes you feel!

3. Hear a voice in your mind's ear say powerfully: *YOU ARE CONFIDENT!*

4. As that feeling reaches a peak: step into that giant you and feel that confident power surge through you. Lock this in! Now.

5. With these wonderful feelings inside imagine that confident you doing something that once bothered you very confidently indeed. Take your time to fully experience that... You can take this act as a sign and a signal that: *all you need is within YOU.*

APPENDIX 4: SITUATIONAL CONFIDENCE BOOST.

This can be used for a general confidence boost, or in some specific situation where you need a confidence boost just before a 'performance' etc. Again light trance only: eyes open or closed. Whichever delivers the most intense experience.

1. Imagine performing really well at something from your own point of view. See that in vibrant colours! You *feel so confident* etc. Feel how great that feels - see that positive response you're getting! Take as much time as you need...

2. Now go up a level. Imagine yourself from your own point of view doing even better! You are looking out through your own eyes at that scene! This confidence is just surging through you! It's who you are! It's going great! Everyone is really impressed with your abilities. And it feels amazing! Just get the gist of that...

3. When you're ready! Go up to level 3: the Mastery Level! See through those eyes and hear through those ears of confidence! You feel an amazing level of confidence unlike anything you've yet known. That person/those people you are interacting with are enjoying what you do. You *feel like a winner*. In this state of mind everything goes well! You are great at doing this, people like what you do very much. Seeing their positive responses makes you *feel even more powerfully confident*. Just do what you do! Wonderfully! That's right. Keep these feelings - they are yours, forever!

Printed in Great Britain
by Amazon